DIARY OF A FEMALE GP

A Week in the Life of 'lazy' female GP in the UK

Joni Martins

Version 1
13th of June 2020

Copyright Notice
© 2020 Joni Martins

GP surgeries will be forced to give patients appointments when they want or face funding cuts, Theresa May has announced as she attempts to relieve the pressure on crisis-hit Accident & Emergency units.

The Prime Minister will demand that GP surgeries meet the Government's pledge to open from 8 am to 8 pm seven days a week unless they can prove that there is no demand in their area.

A major package of Government funding will be "contingent" on GPs being able to "demonstrate" that they are offering appointments "when patients want them", ministers will say.

The Telegraph

13 JANUARY 2017

LEGAL DISCLAIMER

This book is based on real life. The names, characters and incidents portrayed in it, although based on real-life, do not relate to real persons, living or dead, events or locations. Any resemblance to actual persons (other than the GP and her family), living or dead, events or localities is entirely coincidental.

This book is dedicated to all those hard-working people in healthcare, whether they are GPs, hospital-related health care workers, practice nurses, healthcare assistants, receptionists or any of the other very many services provided to help us all maintain and improve our health where possible.

FOREWORD

IN JANUARY 2017 the then British Prime Minister Theresa May upset many hard-working General Practitioners (GPs) in the UK. She stated that all GP-surgeries would be required to open from 8 am till 8 pm daily or face cuts in their funding. Mrs May's reasoning for this was that their failure to open during these hours led to A&E departments being overstretched. Her statement, in turn, was by many interpreted as GPs being lazy people, who did not pull their weight.

Quite understandably GPs did not agree with this and there was quite an uproar in the GP medical press. This even gave rise to a writing competition in which GPs were asked to write a letter to Mrs May to ask her for more support for General Practice.

This book shows an insight into the life of one of those 'lazy' GPs, who even dared to work part-time as she also had a family to look after. Although this shows a presentation of real-life General Practice, none of the details regarding patients are identifiable to protect their privacy and maintain confidentiality. Any resemblance to actual persons, living or dead, events or localities is entirely coincidental.

Something which the government at the time also did not consider; was that especially smaller practices would not have the capacity nor the resources to provide all the hours Mrs May felt were necessary.

I'm sure you will all be capable to judge for yourselves whether GPs are really lazy or whether they are as hard-working as they think they are. This book describes an average week in the life of Dr Ellen, a female GP who struggled to find a balance between given her patients her all and not neglecting her role as a housewife and mother of four in the process.

Dr Ellen (not her real name) is a close friend of mine, who has now retired from practice. She has allowed me to put her experiences to paper.

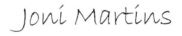

Joni Martins

CONTENTS

CHAPTER 1

Monday, 3:45 am

At a quarter to four on Monday morning, my Fitbit announces the start of another working week. As I open my eyes and become aware it is time to get up again, I stretch and yawn, then hesitantly place my feet on the floor next to the bed. Brr, the house is still cold and a shiver runs down my spine. My husband is still asleep and I try to avoid disturbing him. If only I could stay in bed myself, but work is waiting.

Last night I didn't sleep well. Worries about oversleeping and things I need to do today popping through my head, woke me several times during the night.

On the way to the bathroom, dragging my feet, I pick up my handbag and unplug the charger. As the mobile phone ran out of juice last night, I set it to charge overnight. I leave my bag near the bedroom door and enter the bathroom, turning the light on as I do; still trying to make as little noise as possible. After seeing to my needs, a wash and getting dressed in jeans and a shirt, I get a bowl and cleaning rags to clean the bathrooms. Our home has two bathrooms and a separate toilet and these require cleaning on a daily basis. There are six of us in the house after all.

When we bought the house in 1999 it was a new-built. We enter the house on the middle floor, with a living room to the left and the garage on the left. Upstairs are four bedrooms and two bathrooms. Downstairs is the kitchen, another bedroom, and the back garden.

After cleaning the en-suite, I pick up the bowl and leave the bathroom, then turn off the light. On my way out of the bedroom, I pick up the handbag and laundry left at the bedroom door. This is always a tricky business as the door squeakes and some of the floorboards do too. Avoiding those creaky floorboards best I can, I then move on to the other bathroom, switch on the light and start the cleaning there.

Another ten minutes later, I grab everything, having also replaced the towels with clean ones, and walk downstairs to the toilet. The same process is repeated there and half an hour after waking up, I walk down another flight of stairs to the kitchen.

* * *

Downstairs, I place the bowl in the sink in the utility room, put the laundry in the laundry basket and return to the kitchen.

A quick clean of the worktop, and it is ready for the

next job, baking fresh bread for the family. Baking bread, for me, is stress relief. Although it's a job in itself, it relaxes me and allows me to literally knead away the stresses of the day ahead.

As I set the kettle to boil, I grab the scales and take yeast and butter from the fridge. Next, I collect the flour from the cupboard under the stairs, and no, we don't have Harry Potter living there, only our supplies and the obligatory spiders.

Back in the kitchen, I crumble half a cube of yeast in a measuring jug and add a teaspoon of sugar, then add 250 ml of warm water (half boiling and half cold) and mix this after also adding hot water to my teacup. I place the jug on the scales and add 150 grams of white bread flour and mix again. After putting this to the side until it bubbles, I get a bowl and measure 300 grams of bread flour, usually a mix of white, brown and wholemeal, add 30 grams of butter cut in small pieces and a teaspoon of salt. I mix this mixture until most of the butter has crumbled within the flour. Creating a depression in the middle of this mixture, I pour in the contents of the measuring jug and mix everything together until a smooth dough is formed.

And now it is time for the fun part, the part which can be used for stress relief too. I turn over the bowl and place the dough on the worktop, ready for kneading.

After years of trying and reading about bread-making, I now know kneading it with one hand and folding the dough over itself again and again seventy-five times, gives the best result. Obviously turning the dough around for every new folding action, simply pushing one side to the other.

Now the kneading is also done, I return the dough to the bowl and cover it with a moist tea towel. The dough is left for ten to twenty minutes to rise while I turn my attention to the next task. But first I switch on the oven to allow it to preheat to two hundred and twenty degrees Celsius.

Time to return to the utility room, get the cleaning rag and clean the washing machine, first the little detergent drawer, then the door and the seal. The bin is next on the cleaning list; I remove the bin bag and take it upstairs to the wheelie bin in the garage, taking some of the recycling up with me at the same time. When I return to the utility room again, I clean the bin on the outside, place a new bin bag inside and then clean the lid. I grab the larger cleaning cloth and, just like I cleaned the bathroom and toilet floors earlier, I start mopping the kitchen and utility room floors. As this is something I do on a daily basis, I have learned that I can manage this in the same time the dough needs to rest.

I return to the dough now, turn it onto the worktop again and knead it as before. Back into the bowl it goes again for the second resting period, while I unpack the dishwasher, clean any of the dishes needing to be done by hand and clean the worktops and the table again. Once this is done, I set the table for breakfast and place the lunchboxes next to plates and bowls.

The dough still needs to rest for another few minutes and while I wait for it to be ready for its next action, I get the laundry from the dryer. After placing the laundry into a basket, I place the basket on top of the stove, and grab the ironing board and iron. My next job of the day is folding and ironing the clean laundry. I have time to fold a few clothes before it is time to shape the dough into bread rolls.

To form the dough in bread rolls, I cut the dough in eight more or less equal-sized pieces. These are one by one formed into bread rolls. Starting at six and twelve o'clock, I grab the edges and fold them to the middle, then three and nine, two and seven, and eleven and five. I repeat this another time, roll them in my hands to round the edges a little and place them with the folded side downwards on a baking tray. The moist tea towel goes over the top again and I leave them for another ten minutes while continuing the folding.

When I finish the folding, I switch on the iron and

place the bread rolls, minus tea towel obviously, in the oven for twenty minutes. A glance at the clock tells me it is twenty to five, which means they should be ready in time for my husband coming downstairs.

While ironing the clothes, I watch the BBC news and get alerted to yet another scare. Statins, otherwise known as cholesterol tablets, have been linked to a rise in blood sugar levels. This will be reason enough for several high-risk patients to either stop the statins without asking or informing their doctor or request an emergency appointment to discuss this news further. The week ahead is likely to be a busy one.

After I finish the ironing and place the clean laundry in the basket ready for taking upstairs and putting away, I put away the iron and ironing board.

Great timing; the oven beeps; the bread is also ready. I remove the bread from the oven and leave it on the stove to cool a little. Next, I turn the kettle on and grab a cup for Martin to get his coffee ready. Already I hear the floorboards creak in our bedroom. Martin is up and getting ready for his workday.

My husband is also a GP and works in a different practice. Every Monday and Friday he leaves at half-past five to start surgery at seven. Although the journey does not take long, he prefers to arrive at work early and take care of paperwork before surgery starts.

We are quite alike in that really.

As soon as the bread rolls have sufficiently cooled, I grab two and cut them open, add cheese and place them in Martin's lunchbox. Good, all is ready for him now.

* * *

Around a quarter past five Martin joins me in the kitchen, we hug and say good morning and follow the news while drinking our coffee and tea. Martin does not usually eat breakfast before work even though everyone always mentions breakfast is the most important meal of the day.

This time early in the morning is part of 'our' time. The children are still asleep and I put my arms around him while we watch the news together. I really lucked out with this guy.

The news repeats the statin story and Martin turns towards me, "Well, we know what the theme will be this week." I nod and Martin continues, "I actually read that story in the BMJ over the weekend." The British Medical Journal or BMJ is one of the medical journals that come through the mail on a weekly basis in our house. "There is indeed a slight rise in blood sugar levels during statin use in patients already at risk of developing diabetes. However, the risk of developing diabetes, as a result, is far lower than the risk of having a heart attack or stroke if the statin is stopped in high-risk patients."

I read the same information in a different medical journal online in the weekend myself. At least we now will be able to advise the patients properly and inform them of the actual risks.

* * *

Soon, the weather forecast starts and once it finishes, Martin picks up the lunchbox and leaves the kitchen. As I follow him upstairs, I pick up the basket of laundry. After collecting his work bag and coat from the living room - it always annoys me Martin doesn't put his coat on the coat rack in the hallway - he unlocks the front door and we say goodbye. For Martin, it is time to leave for work. A hug, a kiss and an "I'll see you later, have a good day at work" and he is off.

Then I continue to go upstairs and put the clean laundry away. I leave the clothes for the kids outside their doors, I don't want to disturb them. Half past five is a little early to wake them up.

* * *

After putting the laundry away, I strip our bed and put new covers on. Next I place the bedding in the now empty basket and use the bathroom again before returning downstairs. I place the laundry in the washing machine and turn it on. A quick twenty-minute cycle to allow me to put it in the dryer, or if the weather is right to hang it outside, before my workday. It also allows me to put another load of washing in before I need to leave for work.

* * *

The next job is to dust the house. Starting in the kitchen and working my way up, the dusting usually takes half an hour. By now it is six and the eldest and the middle son, we have three sons and a daughter, come to the kitchen to eat breakfast. Their lunchboxes and lunches are already waiting for them.

I turn towards Archie and Adam, "Morning, did you sleep well?"

As I have been up for over two hours, I am already wide awake. Not so for the middle son Adam, his mood leaves something to be desired at this time of day, "Grr, shut up."

Better not to respond and just leave Adam to it. Archie murmurs and nods to let me know he slept well.

This is the part of a GP's life people don't get to see.

Underneath we are no different; we also have the stresses of a family and housework to cope with.

* * *

Again, I make my way back to the cupboard under the stairs and now collect the vacuum cleaner and return the feather duster. Although our daughter hates me for using the vaccuum cleaner at this time of day, if I want to have any chance of keeping on top of the housework and maintain a career, I'll just need to get on with it. Another half an hour of cleaning and this job is also behind me. By now, I'm quite sweaty and desperately need a shower but first I need to return the vaccuum cleaner to the cupboard.

At half-past six our daughter also comes down for her breakfast and, as expected, Amy is not pleased with me. "Couldn't you have done that a little later? You woke me up again."

"Sorry sweetheart but it needs to be done." I turn around and start to make a shopping list. Monday mornings are also used to get the weekly shop in.

* * *

When she returns to her bedroom to rest for a while before getting ready for school, I run upstairs for a quick shower and to get dressed for the day ahead. On Monday I work a few hours for Martin as they don't have a female GP available. This way the patients are given a slight choice. Two hours is not a lot, but it is better than no choice at all.

Phew, after the rush of the morning cleaning session, the shower is a welcome event. A short resting point in an otherwise busy morning.

* * *

At seven, I return to the kitchen with another load of washing. The washing machine has finished with the bedding and I put this in the dryer, then turn on the next load of washing.

With that job also behind me, I now grab my work laptop and start work.

Although I don't work at my surgery on a Monday, I still like to keep up with the paperwork as much as possible. One of my pet hates is to come into work on a Tuesday to find a pile of paperwork waiting for me. It stresses me out and ruins my day.

So, instead, I take out my laptop on a Monday, check any new pathology results, that is blood tests, urine cultures, sputum cultures, smears etc, and deal with those that I can complete at home. For any prescriptions that are required based on the results, like antibiotics, I check on the patient's notes to ensure they have not already been issued in my absence and then issue those still needing to be issued. From the distance, I am of course not able to sign the prescriptions, unless they are electronic ones, but I send a task to the receptionists to inform the patient of the result and to print off the prescription ready for me to sign the next day.

Results that require a patient to consult a doctor, are sent as a task to the receptionists to invite the patient to see the doctor for the results. The task includes a timeframe where appropriate. Blood results relating to diabetic patients are checked, remarks added and then forwarded to the diabetic nurse as she will see them in the near future, anyway.

By now it is half-past seven and time to wake our youngest son. Alex is still in primary school and leaves later than the other three. Archie, Amy and Adam should soon leave to catch the bus to school too. While waking the youngest, I also check in on them to make sure they haven't fallen asleep again.

When the youngest is out of bed, I return to the kitchen and work.

Now it's time to look at the task list. Amazingly, tasks have come in since I last checked on Friday afternoon. These I also clear as far as possible and then focus my attention on the scanned letters next. A few letters were added to my inbox since Friday afternoon too and I read and deal with these as far as possible. There are a few letters I can only act on at the surgery and they will need to wait until tomorrow.

Archie's door creaks as he gets out of his room and starts to climb the stairs. The noise of the toilet flushing upstairs, followed by footsteps coming down the stairs, reaches me. The voices of Archie and Amy reach me in the kitchen as they tell Adam to get a move on. His irritated response follows. I shout a "Have a good day at school" up to them and not long after hear the front door open and close. They have left for school.

By now, Alex has finished his breakfast and returns upstairs to get dressed while I continue the paperwork. There are a few electronic prescriptions waiting in my inbox to be signed now too.

Wait? Why are they there? Everyone at work is aware I do not work on Friday afternoon or Monday and should not get any prescriptions assigned to me during that time.

Still, there are thirty-five prescriptions waiting for me. They are lucky I check work even on the days I don't work or they could have expected patient complaints. Complaints that prescriptions were not dealt with in the time we promise, within 48 hours on working days.

I check the time, eight already. In the bottom of the computer screen, I notice even more tasks have been assigned to me. There are still twenty minutes before I need to leave for the school run. For the second time today, I open the task screen and check the new tasks received and complete them. Five minutes later, an instant message pops up on the screen. "Are you at it again Dr Ellen?" Michelle always likes to tell me off for working too much.

"You know me, hate to leave things till tomorrow when they can be done today."

Five minutes later another instant message pops up. "Sorry to bother you, but Dr K has not arrived yet. Can you look at the second ring-back please? Not sure if it needs urgent action."

Patricia really should know better than to pass that to me on my days off. She has been told about this time and time again, but still feels too insecure to leave it as it is. Still, I can't ignore a request like this and check the ring-back.

What I find leaves me even more annoyed. Patricia really should have known better. A 56-year-old gentleman with known heart problems has central chest pain and is sweaty and breathless. I immediately send an instant message back to her to advise the patient to call 999 straight away or to call 999 for him, then enter the advice on the notes. These are the symptoms of a possible heart attack and our receptionists know to advise patients of this immediately.

A few minutes later an instant message pops up, "Thanks Dr Ellen, the patient will phone 999, his wife is with him."

I breathe a sigh of relief and hope against hope she will take the right action if next faced with this problem.

* * *

By now it's twenty-five past eight, five minutes later than planned. I log off, take the smart card from the laptop and climb the stairs warning Alex it's time to leave, then use the bathroom before we leave for school. At this time of the day, there is usually heavy traffic on the route to school and it takes nearly half an hour to arrive.

Today, we are lucky to find a parking spot, get out of the car and hurry to the playground. Alex finds his friends and plays for a moment while I talk with some of the other parents and we wait for the teachers to arrive and take the kids inside.

"Off to work again today, Ellen?" asks one of the mums.

"Yes, a quick trip to the shops and then it's time to go to work again. How about you?"

"Oh, I just need to get back to the housework. I'm back at work tomorrow."

We return to the car park together, say goodbye and I set off for the weekly shop.

* * *

At ten past nine, I enter the shop and run through it collecting food and supplies for the working week ahead. The shopping trip usually takes about half an hour and when I have paid and put the shopping in the boot of the car, I return home again. If work isn't too bad on Thursday, I'll do another trip on the way home, otherwise Alex will just need to come with me as I get the shopping in on Friday afternoon. But hopefully, Alex will not have to suffer through this. Like most kids, he does not enjoy shopping trips. Then again, nor do I.

* * *

Just after half-past nine, I return home and put the

shopping away. This takes about ten minutes. By now the dryer has finished and I take the bedding out and refill it with the next load of washing. A brief look at the clock tells me it is already a quarter to ten now and time to get ready for work.

 Although the workday still has to start, I already feel tired.

CHAPTER 2

Monday, 9:50 am

Another visit to the bathroom, then I brush my teeth, and I apply a little lipstick and eyeshadow. Next, I brush my hair once more, walk downstairs to get my work bag and coat and grab my keys. The entire process takes no more than ten minutes and I'm ready to leave. All ready for the day ahead.

* * *

After unlocking the front door, I rush to the alarm and arm it as no one will be in the house for the next few hours. Then I get out, lock the door and place my bag in the boot of the car. Now it is time for the half an hour journey to my husband's work.

* * *

On the drive to work, the radio once again reminds me of the story on the news today and I wonder how many patients will come to discuss this today. The majority of the patients I see are however women with female problems and children. I hope I can at least find a parking space today. The parking lot is small for the size of the building and it is not unusual to need to wait until a space becomes available. This is also the reason I leave for work an hour before I'm due to be there. Even if the journey only takes half an hour.

* * *

Although the surgery today does not start until eleven, I like to arrive well before time. Today I am in luck and a parking space is available immediately. I park the car, get my back and make my way inside. When I reach reception, I greet Siobhan, who is manning the station this morning. She is a friendly and chatty person and always has a story to tell. Five minutes later we move to the room I'll be using today and Siobhan unlocks the door, "There you go, Dr Ellen, it's all set for you."

The computer has already been switched on and I log in, checking the appointment list for today. Although the first patient is booked in for eleven, I notice she has already arrived. A name I am now familiar with as she returns every three months for a pessary change. As far as I am concerned, there is no need to wait till eleven to call her in, so instead, I use the bathroom, then return to the waiting area to collect the first patient of the day. Starting early may even help me run on time today.

One of my pet hates, and I'm sure of my patients too, is to run behind schedule and keep patients waiting. It makes me feel like I'm not good enough, a hang-up from my youth when my dad made it clear he felt I wasn't. But that is behind me now and it's time to put that aside and start the workday.

CHAPTER 3

Monday, 10:30 am

Mary is a sixty-three-year-old lady, who has seen me every three months for the last year for a ring pessary change. After collecting her from the waiting room we stroll to the consulting room together.

"A bit wet this morning, don't you think?" Mary tries to strike up a conversation. It indeed was rather wet this morning and I agree with her.

We enter the room and take a seat, "Is it that time again already?" I ask.

Mary nods and produces the ring pessary, "Here you go doctor, nice and warm as you advised."

The ring pessaries are made of a PVC like material and can be rather stiff when cold. One way to ensure they are warm and therefore soft, is to store the pack in your bra.

Mary stands up and moves to the bed, a routine well established by now.

"Are you still happy with the pessary or do you

experience any problems with it?"

"Oh, no doctor, it really works and I'm happy with it. I have no more problems with losing urine or accidents and, as you said, it is much easier than surgery. At least there is no waiting time and no long recovery after."

By now Mary is ready and waiting behind the curtain surrounding the bed. I join her and put on the gloves, take out the tube of K-Y-jelly and open the packet containing the new ring pessary. As the name indicates, the pessary resembles a ring, albeit larger than what you would put on your finger. After applying the jelly to it and rubbing it all over the pessary with my gloved finger, I first remove the old pessary and then insert the new one. This is all done within a matter of minutes and I glance at Mary's face when it is finished, "All done, does that feel okay?"

"Yes, thank you, doctor," a smile rests on Mary's lips as I leave her to get dressed and discard the old pessary in the clinical waste bin. While I enter the details on the notes, Mary gets dressed and we both finish around the same time.

"So, I'll see you in another three months."

We say goodbye and Mary leaves.

* * *

When Mary leaves at ten past eleven, the second patient for today is already waiting. Although this patient was not due until twenty past eleven, I again collect her early.

Ellie is a five-month-old girl accompanied by her maternal grandmother. Grandma's hair looks unkempt and stains cover her navy dress. I'm sure there are chocolate finger prints on the chest area. The elegant dress does not fit with how grandma presents.

Ellie has a cough which started last night and grandma is adamant Ellie needs antibiotics. When I ask grandma what I can do for Ellie, she is quick to point this out, "Ellie has a really nasty cough doctor. You need to give her some antibiotics to get rid of it."

Rather than get in an argument with grandma straight away, I nod, "Okay, let's check Ellie first." I check her ears and throat, the glands in her neck and they are all normal. Next, I listen to Ellie's chest and that is clear, no sign of infection. Her temperature is only 37.2, which is normal and grandma informs me she has had no paracetamol or ibuprofen.

As far as all the findings indicate, antibiotics are not required and I carefully explain this to grandma.

"Everything seems okay at the moment. There is no indication that Ellie has a bacterial infection and I am afraid antibiotics do not work for viral infections and colds. At the moment I would advise to observe Ellie closely and if she does not improve or if anything changes or gets worse, to seek medical attention again."

Grandma does not look happy, "But doctor, the daughter of my neighbour had exactly the same thing and needed antibiotics. Macey was better after a few days. Surely you can give Ellie some as well?" her eyes narrow as she gazes at me, "Or is this about money again? Are we not good enough to get expensive medication?"

Again I try to explain how antibiotics are not helpful in this situation and grandma leaves with Ellie in her arms. I am not convinced grandma believed my explanation, but it would be bad practice to prescribe antibiotics when they are not needed. This could potentially lead to even more severe problems. Apart from the side effects antibiotics can have, using them when they are not required also leads to the development of bugs which are no longer sensitive to the antibiotics we use. No, I really shouldn't prescribe antibiotics unless they are clinically indicated.

* * *

After entering Ellie's details on her record in detail, it is always possible grandma will complain later, I close the record and return to the appointment screen. It is important to put full details of what occurred and the findings of the examination down on the notes in case anything goes wrong later.

The third patient, a thirty-five-year-old man, has arrived, and I collect him ten minutes before his appointment time. The way back to the consultation room progresses slow. Mark's left lower leg is in a plaster and he limps on crutches.

"So, what can I do for you today?" Never assume a patient comes to see you for a reason which stares you in the face. He could suffer from a sore throat and seek medical attention for that.

Mark looks up, "Well doctor, I need to have a sick note for work please."

He tells me how he jumped over a wall four weeks ago, twisted his left ankle and broke it in the process. Mark has now been in plaster for four weeks and won't visit the consultant for another two weeks. He needs to have another note to cover those two weeks.

This is a relatively easy request and the notes confirm Mark indeed fractured his left ankle. Next, I fill the fit note and sign it, then hand it to Mark. As he leaves the room, I enter the details on his notes and return to the appointment screen.

* * *

By now I am running fifteen minutes ahead of schedule and my next patient has not arrived yet. For just such occasions where there is time not filled with seeing patients, I bring my Kindle and I read for a moment while keeping an eye on the appointment screen. This only happens at my husband's work where I only see patients and am not involved with actioning with results, letters, routine prescriptions and tasks. I don't have time to do this at my own surgery.

Five minutes before her scheduled appointment, my fourth patient arrives, a twenty-nine-year-old woman. As I return to the waiting area to collect her, screaming kid's voices reach me from the waiting area.

Shelly is the mother of three young children, Libby who is three months old, Bobby who is eighteen months old and Tilly who is five and currently in school. Her partner and the dad to her children left her two months ago for another woman and now she is left taking care of three active children. The pain of Sam's betrayal and the loss of the relationship weigh heavy on Shelly, who is depressed and cries a lot. As her parents have retired to Spain and her sister lives thirty miles away and is too busy with her own family and career, Shelly is rather isolated and lonely.

Sam's parents live around the corner from her and

they help where they can. However, they are not supportive and tell her she is a failure as a mother and should hand over custody of the children to their son.

Shelly cries the entire consultation and I listen and comfort as best I can while also keeping an eye on her eighteen-month-old. Bobby crawls through the room, under the desk and opens cupboards and drawers. Shelly is too distraught to notice, and it is on me to keep him safe. Although she calls out to him at times, "Bobby, don't do that" and "That is naughty", he takes no notice of her.

"I'm just a failure doctor. Maybe Sam's parents are right and I should just let him have the kids. I'm no use as a mother to them."

Shelly's crying intensified again.

"What would you like to happen, Shelly? Do you really believe they are better off with Sam?"

Tearful eyes meet mine, "I don't know doctor. But I don't want to lose my children. Before Sam left me, I was a good mum."

Again she dissolves in a flood of tears. Then she sits up a little straighter, "No, I'm not going to let this bring me down. I am a good mum and it was Sam who left us. But I do need some help, is there anything you can suggest?"

We discuss Shelly's symptoms a while longer and

after ensuring the kids are safe in her presence and Shelly is not suicidal, I hand her a leaflet for self-referral to the local mental health services to receive counselling. She appears a little less depressed when she leaves and I ask her to come and see us to talk whenever she feels the need to.

Unfortunately this consultation has taken twenty minutes and I now run five minutes behind.

* * *

The fifth patient today is 56-year-old Brian, a patient known with COPD, or chronic obstructive pulmonary disease. Something that used to be called chronic bronchitis in the past. While we slowly move towards the consultation room, I can hear the wheezing and the ruttles as Brian coughs.

"So, what can I do for you today?" I have a fair idea, but it is wrong to assume. This might be his normal state.

"Well doctor, I have had this cough for the last week and it is not getting any better."

When I enquire after the colour of the sputum, Brian tells me the phlegm is green, and he feels more breathless than usual.

As I listen to Brian's chest, there are crackles present on the right side and the wheezing can be heard on both lungs. His oxygen levels are 95% which are quite good. I go through his notes and ask Brian as well to ensure he has no allergies. A prescription is done for a week of antibiotics and I ask him whether he still smokes.

"Yes doctor, I'm afraid so. I've tried to stop in the past, but not been successful."

After explaining the link between smoking and COPD and the decline of COPD and asking him to seek medical attention if his symptoms do not improve after a few days or if they get worse, Brian leaves again with a promise to try smoking cessation again.

* * *

When the sixth patient of today enters my room, I'm still running five minutes behind. Angela is a twenty-one-year-old woman who attends to request the contraceptive pill. She has spoken to her friends who recommend the combined pill as this also regulates their periods. Angela's periods are a little irregular, she never knows if her cycle will be 26 or 28 days and would like to have a more reliable prediction of her periods. Actually, periods like Angela's are still considered regular, but there is no need to upset Angela by telling her this.

"Before we can decide which contraceptive option is

the best one for you, I need to ask you a few questions and check a few things if that is alright?"

Angela nods.

When I double-check she has no personal history of blood clots or of migraines, Angela confirms she has not.

"Do you smoke?"

"Not much," she turns her gaze down to her lap, an indication it may be more than she admits to.

"How much is not much?"

"Well, about twenty a day, but that is not much, right?"

Sorry, I can't agree with Angela. Twenty is a lot, and the combined pill is not recommended for smokers. If she had only smoked five a day at most, this might be overlooked, but with the number of cigarettes she smokes every day the risk of blood clots rises to an unacceptable level and I inform Angela of this. Then I grab the cuff of the blood pressure monitor.

"I'll also need to check your blood pressure."

Again, her blood pressure is a little on the high side and this increases the risk even further.

Next Angela steps on the scales and my suspicions she is obese are confirmed. No, the combined pill definitely is not the right option for this young lady.

"Okay. There are a few things we need to consider.

Although the combined pill makes periods more regular, your periods are already fairly regular. The next problem is that if a woman smokes, is overweight and has a raised blood pressure all these factors separately increase the risk of forming blood clots while on the combined pill. It is therefore not recommended to give you the combined pill."

Angela's face clouds over.

"However, there are other options we can consider. You could try the mini pill. This only contains one hormone rather than two and needs to be taken every day, so no break week as with the combined pill. You could also consider the injection, which needs to be given every twelve weeks into your buttocks and the majority of women have no periods on that. Or you could consider the implant which lasts you for three years. Further options would be the coil which lasts for five years. And there is, of course, the possibility of using condoms. They are not as reliable as the other options, but I would recommend using them with any of the other forms of contraception to protect you from sexually transmitted disease too."

Angela nods, but obviously is not very happy, "So you won't give me the combined pill?"

I shake my head, "No, I'm sorry, the combined pill would not be a safe option for you."

"Would you be able to give me the implant today?"

Again I shake my head, "Sorry, I'm afraid none of the doctors at this surgery is currently trained for the implant. I can, however, give you the details of where you can have that done if you wish. In the meantime, you could use the minipill and at least be covered."

Angela nods, "So when should I start taking the pill?"

Now I tell her to take the pill from the first day of her period and to take it every day around the same time. This is followed by an explanation of what factors can influence the effectiveness of the pill. For instance, if she would suffer from vomiting or diarrhoea, she might not absorb the pill and therefore it might not be effective. If she forgot the pill, the same thing would apply.

Angela nods again, I hand her the prescription and advise her to return after three months to discuss if it suits her unless she has changed to the implant instead.

When the door closes behind Angela, it is a quarter past twelve.

* * *

By now, my seventh patient has arrived and I collect him from the waiting area.

Tom is a twenty-seven-year-old man, who sustained

a back injury while lifting plant pots in the garden and pulled his back. Although his back has improved a lot over the last two weeks and Tom is desperate to return to work, his back still gives him the odd twinge. Tom has tried to lift his two-year-old daughter, but this still caused him considerable discomfort and he suffered for two days after.

Tom works in a warehouse and there is a lot of heavy lifting involved. He has spoken to his boss, who has promised he can go on light duties for a period of time provided he gets a note from the doctor.

After examining Tom's back to ensure nothing was missed, I hand him a fit note for amended duties, heavy lifting is to be avoided for the next two weeks.

When he leaves, I let out a relieved sigh. I have caught up again.

* * *

Next is a ten-year-old girl who attends with her mother. Amy has had cold symptoms for the last four days and still has a snotty nose and a cough. For the last two days, she has also suffered from an earache in her right ear and this worsened over time.

Although Amy has been to school this morning, mum has taken her out of school for the appointment. This appointment conveniently falls in Amy's lunch break.

"Okay Amy, so which one is the naughty ear?" She points at her right ear and her expression is rather thunder-like. Tears brim in her eyes as she bites on her finger.

Grabbing the otoscope, that thing we stick in ears to check them, I first look in her left ear,

"It is her other ear doctor," Mum watches disapprovingly.

"I know, that's why I checked the other one first." Then I check the right ear. The right eardrum is a very angry red. When I check her glands, the one underneath that ear is noticeably swollen, but several glands in her neck are also swollen as evidence of the cold Amy suffers from. As though the snotty nose had not given that away yet. Her throat looks fine and when I listen to her chest, this is clear as well.

All through the examination, I inform Amy and her mum of my findings to keep them up to date. After checking her temperature this is only 37.4, but mum informs me Amy had some paracetamol before coming to the surgery.

With the ear infection confirmed, I hand Amy the prescription. She is now smiling and proud to be given the responsibility of carrying the piece of paper that is her prescription.

"Can she go back to school?"

Yes, if Amy is well enough in herself and school is happy with her taking antibiotics in school, there is no reason why Amy should be kept home. The usual advice to seek medical attention if she does not improve or if she gets worse follows.

As Amy leaves the room, she is skipping, mum rushing to keep up with her.

* * *

Now it is time to see the ninth patient. Six-year-old Billy comes in with his dad, "Doctor, Billy has a painful tiddles."

Tiddles? Well, patients give all kinds of funny names to the penis. They brought a urine sample, but when I check that, it is clear. No sign of a urine infection.

"Can I have a look, Billy?"

Billy crosses his arms and turns around, stamping his feet at the same time, "NO!"

Dad turns him around again, "Come on Billy, the doctor can only help if you let her have a look."

"NO!"

I turn towards Billy, "How about you climb onto that bed there and show me where it hurts?"

His eyebrows relax a little.

"You show me and I look but won't touch."

Billy bites on his lip, then nods and climbs onto the

bed. Dad releases a sigh.

When I examine the offending article, the foreskin is crimson and a pussy discharge seems to sit just underneath.

"Okay, that is all I needed to do, Billy. You can put your trousers back up again and get off the bed again."

He pulls his trousers back up but remains on the bed, arms crossed.

As I turn to dad, I start to explain, "Billy has an infection of his foreskin. The fancy term for that is balanitis. It can easily be treated with antibiotics."

When I prepare the prescription, having checked with dad Billy has no known allergies, Billy is still on the couch.

Dad turns to Billy with the prescription in his hand, "Time to go Billy."

"Don't wanna." After dad's insistence, they leave and it is time for my next patient.

* * *

Now, it's Dorothy's turn. She is fifty-five and has a painful right knee. This knee has caused her some trouble on and off over the last year but has become worse over the last two months. It aches all the time, appears stiff and causes problems when she climbs stairs. Taking her dogs out has also become a struggle, especially on uneven terrain. Dorothy denies any history of trauma and when I examine her knee, there is no swelling, redness and it does not feel hot. The joint is, however, rather knobbly looking.

"Well Dorothy, it appears you have started with osteoarthritis, your knee shows signs of wear and tear. This does not mean you need to stop using it. Quite the contrary, the problem tends to worsen quicker if you rest it while it behaves for longer if you keep moving. If the pain is bad enough, you can take pain relief for it."

"Do I need a knee replacement?" Dorothy's gaze is troubled.

I reassure Dorothy that she does not yet need a knee replacement and that this should be delayed for as long as possible. In general knee replacements should not be done before the patient is sixty-five. Replacement joints often only last 10-15 years and a second replacement is possible but difficult. A third replacement often is not possible.

Dorothy nods, "Can I have a X-ray to make sure?"

At her request, I fill out an X-ray form and ask her to take it to reception with her. The reception staff will then arrange this further for her. Perhaps I should have declined her request forn an X-ray, there is no real indication for this in the early stages of osteoarthritis but Dorothy would likely have been unhappy if I had.

* * *

Finally, it is time for the last patient for today. Yes, Mondays are generally the easy days. Only two hours of surgery.

The last patient has not arrived yet and I read a moment in case he arrives late. In general, I'll wait up to twenty minutes for patients to arrive and if they still haven't arrived, I will leave. That should give them plenty of time.

Helen arrives five minutes late. She is a forty-two-year-old lady and has discovered a lump in her left breast a week ago. Initially, she didn't want to bother anyone with it, convinced it would be nothing. The lump is, however, still present and after reading an article in a magazine she is getting concerned. Still, she apologises for bothering me for something that is probably nothing and I reassure her it is always best to make sure.

Helen takes off her top and bra and I try to warm my hands. They are usually freezing cold and I don't want to cause any more distress than needed.

"My hands may be a little cold. Now, I will first check the right breast. Every woman is different, and it is always good to be able to compare to what is normal in that woman."

As I move my hands over her right breast to examine it, I ask Helen where in her menstrual cycle she is at the moment. Apparently, she is due in a week which explains the lumpiness in the right breast. No distinct lumps, only normal breast tissue. I move to her left breast and repeat the examination on the left side. On the left upper part of her breast, an irregular and hard lump can be felt. The lump is around 2 cm in diameter, but as mentioned irregularly shaped. This is not a good sign.

"Is this where you found the lump?"

Helen nods, and I check her armpits, above her collarbones and around her chestbone for signs of swollen glands. I'm not convinced there isn't a small gland to be found in her left armpit.

After Helen dresses again, we sit down and I explain the findings.

"There is indeed a lump in your left breast. Although I can't be certain, it could be a nasty lump and you were right to have it checked. What I think we should do, is send off a referral to the breast surgeon to have it investigated. They will then be able to find out what it is and what needs to be done next if anything."

"Do you think it is cancer doctor?"

"I can't be certain at the moment, but that is a possibility. The referral I will send is a two-week wait referral, which means you should be seen at the hospital within two weeks. That way you should soon learn more."

"So you think it is cancer?"

"I don't know Helen, but it is possible, and that is why we need to investigate the lump further. When we find out what we are dealing with, we can act accordingly. For now, we have insufficient information to say whether the lump is or whether it is not cancer. The referral is needed to exclude that as a possibility."

While Helen still tries to come to terms with what I told her, I fill in the two-week referral form and hand it to her to take to reception and arrange the appointment at the breast clinic.

I hope I prepared Helen sufficiently for the outcome of the investigations without taking all hope away. Unfortunately, I'm 99% certain Helen indeed has breast cancer, possibly even with spread to the lymph nodes in her armpit. Still, I hope I'm wrong.

CHAPTER 4

Monday, 1:15 pm

Twenty minutes after Helen's arrival, I close down the computer, collect my things and pay a visit to the bathroom. I return to the room to pick up my bag and stride to the reception. Ellen has joined Siobhan in reception for the afternoon.

"Is that everything for today?"

They both nod, "Yes, all done."

After double checking the referral and X-ray form have been dealt with, I turn around to leave. Martin joins us in the reception area at this time, "Leaving?"

"Yes, I was just about to go." After updating him about the last patient, the letter will probably end up in his tray after she has been seen at the hospital, I say goodbye to everyone and leave to go home, "See you next week, ladies!" and add to Martin, "See you tonight. Don't work too hard."

Although I would love to kiss him goodbye, it would not be professional to do so. We are at work, after all.

* * *

When I return home, I put down my bag and move upstairs to change into jeans and a shirt. The formal dress and jacket I reserve for work, the jeans and shirt for housework. As the last patient arrived late and took longer, it is already close to two when I arrive in the kitchen. I grab one of the bread rolls I baked this morning and put cheese on it, boil the kettle and grab a cup-a-soup. Then I return to the kitchen table and turn on my work laptop.

While eating my lunch, I log onto the computer, check work e-mails and log onto the clinical system again.

* * *

More results have arrived in my in-box and I check those first. Fortunately, you can order the results into normal, abnormal and undetermined results as the laboratory has already partially made that decision for us. First, I tackle the normal results, making sure they indeed are normal and file them in the patient's notes. Then I turn my attention to the abnormal results. At this point, I need to send tasks for action to the receptionists and I check all the results for that patient before filing the initial abnormal result I opened. Hopefully, this will avoid unnecessary duplication of work by the receptionists and allow them to contact a patient once rather than several times with different results. It does not fully guarantee this though. Some results may not arrive until the next day, but I try to limit duplication as much as I can.

Once all results are cleared, I turn my attention to the notifications. These are internal e-mails within the clinical system. Patricia has sent me a message to inform me she has already started on the prescriptions for me. Hang on, I don't work on Monday. At least not at my own surgery.

Apparently, a lot of prescription requests have arrived today and Dr K is the only partner in. Dr P is on holiday at the moment and the locums do not deal with repeat prescriptions, results, letters, tasks and visits. With that in mind, it is probably fair enough Patricia has already assigned prescriptions to me today. Still, I'm still not really happy and I wonder how many prescriptions will be waiting in a box for signing when I arrive at work tomorrow.

Next, I check tomorrow's appointment screen. If Dr P is on holiday at the moment, chances are I will be on my own with locums tomorrow. That is, provided the practice manager has been successful in getting locums to cover.

As suspected, I am the only partner scheduled to work

tomorrow. This also means, I'll be the on-call doctor, the doctor to deal with all emergencies to pop up during the day. And to cope with any non-emergencies that patients consider to be an emergency. Only one locum has been booked in, and for two hours in the morning only. That is going to be fun, or more likely, that is not going to be fun.

By the time I have checked this, it is a quarter to three and time to log off and get ready for the school run.

* * *

Although the school does not finish till half-past three, I still leave before three. Parking near the school is always a nightmare even if there is a parking lot at the church and one at the nearby community centre. At ten past three, I park the car and get my Kindle from the handbag to read while waiting for school to finish.

Martin and I are lucky. Although we both work and have no family living nearby, childcare is arranged between the two of us well. Martin takes care of the school run on Tuesdays, Thursdays and the Wednesday morning and I do on Mondays, Fridays and Wednesday afternoon.

At twenty-five past three, I put the Kindle back in the handbag and rush to the playground. School will be out soon.

At the moment I'm reading 'The Beauty Shop' by Suzy Henderson. This book is a wartime novel, describing how a surgeon used ground breaking treatments on burn victims in the second world war. Although it's fiction, Suzy has used a lot of historical facts. I love how the author describes the story of love between the pilots and their girls and how the burns sustained in a crash threaten to destroy this relationship. Definitely a book I can recommend for those interested in the second world war, medicine and love.

* * *

When I reach the playground, the mums of some of Alex's friends are also waiting at school. As I join them, we talk about the weather, an upcoming school trip and how work is. Before long the school doors open and children run out accompanied by their teacher. The children running onto the playground are from a different year. They assemble around their teacher and she lets them join their parents one by one when she has made sure the parents have arrived. Another class emerges, soon followed by a third class. After another five minutes, Alex's class also joins the rest on the playground. As he pulls on the teacher's sleeve, he points me out. She nods and lets him go. Soon his friend George also runs up to join his mother.

After making our way to the car and saying goodbye to his friend and his mum, we drive home again.

* * *

We arrive home around four and Alex puts his schoolbag next to the door, ready for tomorrow. He follows me downstairs to the kitchen where I get him a drink and a snack. Alex is a quiet boy. "How was school today?" Some mumbling is all I get in response and I can't work out what he has said. From experience, I know asking him to repeat it will give the same result and only get him annoyed and I let it go for now. If something was wrong, he would tell me. Like his siblings, Alex does not like talking about school. Next, he goes upstairs to his room to play while I log onto the laptop again to return to the work waiting.

I check the tasks and deal with any I can, there are a few acute prescription requests waiting. Patricia has kept her promise. There is nothing acute about these prescriptions. These are prescriptions that are not on the patients' repeat list, but the patient still requests the item. Sometimes the request is appropriate and sometimes it is not. However, every request needs to be looked at, checked as to why the patient received the prescription in the past and we then need to determine whether it is appropriate to re-prescribe or not. This takes more time than repeat prescriptions and it can also be quite tricky. Several of the requests are inappropriate, and I return the task to the receptionists informing them of this so they can tell the patient. Some requests require further assessment and I send a task for the patient to see a doctor to discuss the medication further before it is next issued. Fortunately, most of these appointments can be in routine, the odd one needs to be seen sooner.

The diabetic nurse has sent several tasks for medication changes. This is after I already suggested these changes based on blood results. Hayley discusses the changes with the patient and her task is the way she communicates the outcome of these discussions. There are also some queries about diabetic care and medication problems and a few requests to give a patient more time to achieve a better diabetic control.

Now that the tasks have been completed, I go to the electronic prescribing screen and electronically sign the repeat prescriptions waiting, seventy-eight so far. As soon as I have cleared this in-box, another twelve arrive and I also sign those.

I change to the in-box for letters and order those. All letters relating to patients are scanned on arrival. These letters are read by a receptionist and the medical secretary, both who have been trained to do so. Obviously, patient confidentiality applies to all people working within the practice, not only the doctors and nurses. They collect all new diagnoses and summarise those on the patient's notes to aid us in providing the best possible care to the patients. If any action is requested in the letter or any medication change is noted, they highlight this and put a red flag next to the letter before sending it to the in-box of the doctor who referred the patient initially. With Dr P being on holiday, letters for Dr P are sent to the duty doctor instead. Today that will be Dr K, tomorrow it will be my turn.

Any X-ray results receive a blue flag. Simple clinic letters without changes or need for action receive a yellow flag. I start with the red-flagged letters. If action is required, it is important to deal with those first. Most are easy and can be sorted this afternoon. A few require action I can only take while at the surgery and these have to wait. Next, I check the blue-flagged letters and put a remark on the result. This could be 'normal' or 'normal for this patient' or 'confirms diagnosis already discussed' or 'see a doctor to discuss result'. The receptionist can pass these remarks on to the patient when he or she phones for the result. In the past we used to phone patients if there was an abnormal result and they relied on this. Then, several years ago, an abnormal result arrived a year after the X-ray was taken. Ever since that time, we have asked patients to phone in for the results as this also works as a failsafe. It also warns us if a result has not been received when it should have been. If an abnormal result is received, we still contact the patient about this and in those cases the remark left on the result is accompanied by a task to the receptionists to alert them to this.

Finally all actionable letters have been actioned bar one and I can start reading all the ones carrying a yellow flag. This is now relatively easy and quick and after half an hour I have concluded these too.

* * *

By now it is a quarter to five and I hear the front door open, Archie, Amy and Adam are home from school too. Adam runs into the kitchen, "Mum, mum, can we have crisps?"

I check the time, knowing it must be around five. Martin won't be home till seven, but I usually get tea for the kids ready before he gets home. Still, their appetite is good, and they had a long day. "Okay, you can have one packet of crisps each, but other than drinks, nothing else. It will be teatime soon." When I ask how school was, the usual unintelligible grunts are my answer.

Adam sets off for the cupboard under the stairs and gets crisps for everyone, also throwing a packet next to my laptop. Not fancying a packet of crisps myself, I resolve to put it back in the cupboard later and close down the work laptop. All in-boxes are clear for now and I will finish the rest in the morning.

Now it's time for some relaxation. I get out my personal laptop and turn it on to check on personal e-mails. There are e-mails from medical websites to alert me to new developments and I scan through those to pick out which articles are relevant to general practice and read those. I check through the e-mails received relating to crafting and action any that need actioning. By the time I catch up with all e-mails, it is already half-past five and time to prepare tea for the kids.

* * *

After shutting down the laptop and tidying it away, I switch on the television and grab the potatoes and peel them. Then I get broccoli from the fridge and cut it in florets before placing it in the steamer tray above the potatoes. The loin steak needs seasoning, and afterwards, I cook the meal. With the food on the stove, I now set the table while watching the telly at times.

Half an hour later, I walk to the stairs, "Tea time!" Shortly after Amy, Adam and Alex run down the stairs and Archie emerges from his bedroom. They all sit down at the table and dig into their food, talking to each other about video games while still chewing their food. No matter how often I tell them not to talk with their mouth full, kids will be kids and do as they please. Soon, the plates are empty and they place them in the dishwasher. Even if I need to scour their rooms for dirty laundry, at least they put the plates in the dishwasher.

Adam turns towards me, "Can we have a dessert?"

Did I buy any? I open the fridge and find yoghurt left on a shelf, "Here you go, you can have yoghurt."

"Thanks, mum," and he skips towards the table again.

With the yoghurt eaten too, Alex gets ready to go to bed and the other three get back to do their homework. Adam needs a bit of encouragement at times, his PlayStation is much more interesting than any piece of homework could ever be. Still, he goes upstairs and turns his attention to his homework.

* * *

By now it is close to half-past six and I peel potatoes, cut broccoli and season the loin steaks for Martin and me. The news is on in the background while I work. Martin usually gets home around seven on a Monday and I start cooking tea around half-past six to have it ready when he gets home. Mondays are long days for him. He leaves at half-past five in the morning and returns around seven. This means he will hardly see the kids today. When they get up, he is already at work and when he returns, at least Alex is in bed already.

While I cook tea, I mull over what will happen at work tomorrow. I can already predict it will be busy. How busy remains to be seen, but busy is a certainty. Still, I work with a great team and we should be able to cope.

* * *

At seven, tea is ready, but there is no sign of Martin yet. I have turned off the stove, not wanting to burn the food and have instead placed it in the oven to keep it warm. Ten minutes later, the front door opens, and he arrives. While the sound of his footsteps climbing the stairs reaches the kitchen, I go upstairs to greet him.

Martin is changing into something more comfortable when I enter the bedroom, "That was a long day."

Martin nods, "Yes, I had to do a visit on the way

home. Why they couldn't have requested the visit this morning, I don't know. Instead, they phoned for the visit at five to six."

After giving Martin a quick hug, we move to the kitchen where I place the food on the table. Martin's eyebrows shoot up, "Is that reheated food?" He hates reheated food and refuses to eat anything which has been reheated.

After reassuring him I only kept it warm in the oven, we eat the meal.

"So, how was the rest of your day?"

Martin tells me about how a patient made trouble at reception for the receptionists, leaning over the counter in a threatening manner. At the moment when Martin strolled into the waiting room to collect his next patient, the patient was reaching for the collar on the receptionist's shirt. Only when Martin asked what was going on, did the patient move back a little and did he raise his concerns with Martin. Apparently, the patient demanded a prescription for a tranquiliser would be printed and signed immediately. This patient was experiencing withdrawal effects from the medication he overused and he demanded another supply.

Even when Martin calmly told him he could not give in to that demand, the patient would not back off and demanded a prescription and calling the practice all names under the sun. Only when they threatened to call the police to escort him off the premises, did the patient back off and leave, promising to return for the prescription the next day.

"He is not getting the prescription tomorrow either, it is not due for another two weeks and I am not going to feed his addiction." Martin took another bite from his food, chewed and swallowed, "He knew when he registered at the practice we do not prescribe valium and he would need to cut down and stop. Instead, he has increased the amount he takes and requests more. I have already told the girls he will need to make an appointment before the next prescription is issued."

When we finish the meal, Martin makes his way upstairs to play on the PlayStation for a moment while I clear the table, turn the dishwasher on and then also go to the living room to spend time with my husband. While he shoots and gets shot in the game to reduce his stress levels, I grab the Kindle and read for fifteen minutes. Then it is time to go upstairs and get ready for bed. It is a quarter to eight already and it will be another early day tomorrow.

CHAPTER 5

Tuesday, 3:45 am

Tuesday starts at a quarter to four when the Fitbit buzzes me awake again. Martin is still asleep and I carefully slide out of bed like every weekday morning, taking care not to wake him. With my bag in hand, I make my way to the bathroom to get ready and dressed. Jeans and a shirt will do for now to ensure my work clothes don't get dirty while doing the housework. I already know today will be busy. How could it be any different with only twelve appointments for the locum and eighteen appointments available for booking with me today? The rest of the day will consist of ring-backs and emergencies. Paperwork will probably need to take a backseat.

* * *

As I push the worries regarding the work pressures ahead of me towards the back of my mind, I start the normal ritual of cleaning the bathrooms and it usually takes about twenty minutes to clean all three. Unless, of course, anyone used the bath the day before. In that case, the bath needs cleaning too, and that adds another five minutes. Once the bathrooms are clean again, I continue my way to the kitchen to start on my other daily tasks.

* * *

It is the same story every day; I put the bowl in the sink, then start preparing the dough for the bread rolls. Today I will make white rolls with sesame seeds on top. Making your own bread has the benefit you can pick and choose and add some variation. Sometimes I will make small baguettes instead and the butter will be left out of the recipe in that case. In that case, a tray will also be put in the bottom of the oven before turning it on to 230 degrees Celsius, and a glass of water is added to that tray just before the dough is put in. The resulting burst of steam ensures a nice hard crust.

Again, the washing machine and bin are cleaned, the floor mopped and dishwasher unpacked. When I have cleaned the worktop again, I place the laundry in the washing machine and turn it on, unpack the dryer and start the folding and ironing once more. This is also a daily chore. At the right intervals, I interrupt what I am doing to knead the dough or form the dough into bread rolls or to place the dough in the oven.

Shortly after five, I pack a lunch for the family and take out the work laptop again, and I also get breakfast for myself.

* * *

After I log on to the clinical system, I check any results received overnight and deal with these. This morning there are another seventy-eight waiting for me. There are twelve results requiring a prescription and unfortunately, the patients involved are not registered for electronic prescribing. Instead, I prepare the prescription and click the 'print later' button. When I get into work later, I will check under 'spooled prescriptions' and print them off, sign them and hand them to the receptionists. I already sent a task to inform the receptionists of this and to inform the patient.

Next stop is the notification screen, a few notifications came in late afternoon and I read and action these. There is a message from the practice manager to let me know we will hold a significant event meeting on Thursday. At significant event meetings, anything that has gone wrong, nearly went wrong or could have gone wrong and was avoided, will be discussed.

Another twenty-two letters arrived since I logged off yesterday and I read these and file them. Only three required action, but these will need to wait until I get to the surgery this morning.

Seventeen prescription tasks are waiting and I complete those, fifteen tasks from the diabetic nurse have been added since yesterday evening and I finish those too. A few of these are a request for a change in the repeat prescriptions to improve diabetic control, some are a request to give the patient a little more time to improve their diet and lifestyle.

At six, Adam and Archie enter the kitchen and I look up, "Morning. Did you sleep well?" Archie nods and Adam grunts his answer as they get a bowl of cereal each and meanwhile prepare their lunches for school. My attention returns to the laptop.

The electronic prescription in-box has another forty-eight prescriptions waiting for me to sign and I complete this while checking the time and feeling the pressure of needing to shut down the laptop and get ready for work. It is already five past six and I need to hurry.

* * *

After switching off the laptop and returning it to its case, I put it over my shoulder and add my work bag. Next, I pick up the basket of laundry, Martin's lunch and a cup of coffee and move upstairs to get ready for a busy day ahead. I tidy away the laundry, put Martin's lunch with his work bag and the coffee on his bedside table, and go to the bathroom to change for work.

After applying lipstick and eyeshadow, I change into the dress and jacket for work. I really can't be bothered to make more of an effort than applying those once a day and leave the lipstick and eyeshadow in their spot in the bathroom. No wonder both have lasted at least ten years. Then I slink over to Martin and kiss him before leaving for work, "See you tonight sweetheart, don't work too hard."

Today Martin can stay in bed until seven or half-past seven; he will take Alex to school later. On Tuesday Martin only works until two and is able to pick Alex up from school again after. While I move towards the bedroom door, I notice how Martin turns over and pulls the covers around him again. If only I could nestle in again, preferably with him, but work is waiting.

CHAPTER 6

Tuesday, 6:28 am

A little before half-past six, I leave the house, get to the car and place my bags in the boot. The journey to work takes about half an hour depending on the traffic, but at this time of day, the roads are usually not too bad. Listening to the radio, I notice the sun rising on the horizon. The orange and yellow hues against the blue sky and the white clouds are soothing and I extract all the calm I can from it. Purposefully I contemplate how good life really is. If I don't force myself to do this on a daily basis, the risk of experiencing the doom and gloom so many patients go through is too great.

There are several idiots on the road this morning, people who have a strong belief that the road is theirs and theirs alone and no one else counts. Another car decides to cut in just in front of me and I need to brake to avoid hitting him. Why he did that I don't know, there is plenty of space around us. It is not as though I am one of those people staying in the middle lane on the motorway all the time. At the moment, I am in the nearside lane; a lane which was empty ahead until he cut me off. The next exit is still miles away, so it isn't as though he needed to cut in quick to catch it.

The story I heard on the news yesterday, is again repeated this morning. Further stories of how statins increase the risk of diabetes by increasing blood sugar levels. How many people will panic today and want to speak to me about this? I'm sure I'll find out later.

After I take my exit, I arrive at work ten minutes later. The gate is still locked, I'm the first person to arrive as usual. As I stop the car in front of the gate, I get the keys and open the gate, then get back in the car and drive to the parking space I usually use. After logging the mileage, I get out of the car, grab my bags and move towards the back door. Again I get out the keys and I open the shutter, unlock the back door and switch off the alarm. The back door locks automatically and I move through the hall turning on the lights on the way.

* * *

When I reach my room, I unlock the door, turn on the light and enter. As I unlock the filing cabinet, I place my bags inside for safekeeping. Unfortunately, unwanted guests occasionally will visit the premises and enter places they are not supposed to get near. In today's world, we need to be ever mindful of the risk of thieves.

I turn on the computer, take out my thermos flask to pour myself a cup of tea and get started. It is only a little after seven in the morning at the moment, but at least this gives me an hour until the surgery opens.

A few work-related e-mails have arrived and I check these while waiting for the clinical system to log me on. Further results have arrived, but I first go to the spooled prescriptions and print them off; I can't forget about them if I already dealt with them. I check the new results, another nineteen have arrived, and file them after the appropriate action has been taken where necessary. While waiting for the computer to open one report after the other, I sign the printed prescriptions and then move on to the next result.

Next, I turn my attention to the letters I could only process when at the surgery. A few require a letter to be written to the specialist. One letter has asked us to prescribe a medication which has been red-listed. This means this medication should not be prescribed by a GP but only by a specialist. After writing a letter informing the consultant of this and that we will be unable to prescribe this medication as per his request, I print the letter off and sign it, placing it to the side to take up to the office later.

Another letter is asking for further information on a patient before the hospital will consider seeing the patient. I check the notes and find out a locum has referred the patient and indeed forgotten to provide all the information required. Now it falls to me to remedy this and provide the consultant with all required information. Hopefully, this will not increase the waiting time for the patient to be seen.

By now it is twenty to eight and noises reach me from reception. The first receptionists arrive to set up for the day, open consultation rooms and switch on the computers.

A knock on the door, "Come in."

Michelle pops her head in, "Morning Dr Ellen, did you have a good weekend?"

"Yes, thank you, I had a great time. Just nice and relaxing with the family as I like it."

Her eyebrows furrow, "Today will be a difficult one I think. There are only a few appointments left over."

As I open the appointment screen, I notice only five appointments are left open to book for today.

"Dr K asked for patients from ring-backs yesterday to be booked in today."

That is not quite how it is supposed to be. The majority of our appointments are supposed to be for book on the day only. Doctors are able to overrule this, but only leaving five appointments available to book on the day does not seem quite right.

"Don't worry, it's not your fault. We'll cope as we always do. We're a team, remember?" A sigh threatens to escape as I contemplate how difficult this day is likely to become.

Michelle's gaze is thunderous, "Still, it is not right. They should not leave you to pick up the pieces." Michelle hands me a box of prescriptions, an apologetic expression on her face, "Sorry, these were left for you in reception last night," and she leaves.

Oh joy! Today is really going to be a fabulous day. Yes, I am being sarcastic. The poor receptionists are going to be at the brunt of it all. They will receive all the abuse from patients due to the lack of appointments. And I will need to do all in my power to keep the pressure down as much as possible and keep control of the situation. My head already starts to pound a little, and I drink my tea. It is important to make sure I remain hydrated to avoid headaches as much as possible. A headache would only make today harder than it already is going to be. I will need all my wits about me and a distracting headache would make that difficult.

But, back to work.

While I grab the box with prescriptions, I open the screen where I can find the online prescription requests. This is generally only used by the receptionists, however, as every prescription will land on my desk today anyway, I might as well get rid of those while I can. Again, I sign prescriptions while patient records load, deal with the online prescriptions and sign them electronically or print them off and sign them by hand, sign prescriptions from the box, etc.

At five to eight I have finished the prescriptions and placed them back in the box, the online requested ones added to it.

* * *

As I get up to get ready for the day ahead, I grab the box of prescriptions and saunter to reception. Elaine mans the front desk today. We greet each other and try to encourage each other today will be fine although there are no guarantees it will be and it is far more likely today will be a nightmare.

After I hand Elaine the prescriptions, I climb the stairs, meeting Linda, in the hallway. Linda is our healthcare assistant, and she also does some administrative work for the practice manager. "Sorry, I was unable to get more than one locum for today, Dr Ellen."

I tell her that is okay, I know she has done her best. We'll simply have to cope.

When I get into the office, Michelle is on the phone speaking to a patient. It is only one minute past eight, but already I can detect from her voice that the patient is rather aggressive, "I'm really sorry Mr K, but I have no appointments left for this afternoon. Two appointments are still available for this morning." She holds the phone away from her ear and we can hear him shout through the phone, "Well that's no bloody use now, is it? You are a disgrace, you never have any appointments if I need them," then throws the phone down on her.

No, today's outlook is definitely not a good one.

Libby is on the phone to another patient, "Okay Mrs A, you are booked in with the locum this morning at ten. We'll see you then."

Both girls seem rather downcast. Although I'm not very hopeful for a good day today either, I know I need to pick them up a little, "Don't worry girls, we can do this. We did it before and we'll manage today too. If we only work together like the team we are, we can do this."

I pace to the box my mail gets put into and pick it up, rifling through it and using the bin as a filing system for all junk mail. Next, I march to the bathroom and return to pick up the mail and bring it with me downstairs.

Let the mayhem begin.

* * *

When I arrive back in my room, it is ten past eight. The first patient is booked for half-past eight and has not arrived yet. This leaves me a bit of time to check the ring-backs if any have arrived and go through the mail if possible.

Checking the mail turns out to be an idle hope as six ring-backs arrived already.

At our surgery, we offer any patient who feels their problem is an urgent one requiring attention the same day, the option of having a ring-back by the duty doctor. Today that doctor is me. The receptionist asks basic details, name, address, date of birth, phone number and a brief description of the problem they wish to discuss with the doctor. To have this description at hand helps us to prioritise the right patients where possible. Sometimes the description makes it obvious only a prescription is required, other times it is obvious a patient needs to be seen and sometimes seeing another professional like the pharmacist, is more appropriate.

Before the first patient arrives, I check the ring-backs

and process those I can already.

* * *

The first ring-back of the day is from twenty-one-year-old Krista. Last night she had intercourse with her boyfriend and her condom broke, she requests the morning-after pill.

I pick up the phone and call her. The sooner Krista receives the appropriate treatment, the bigger the chance it will be successful.

"Is that Krista?" She confirms it is. "Are you able to speak at the moment?" Krista again answers in the affirmative. Great. It is always important to make sure the patient is able to speak due to confidentiality. Perhaps she does not want her parents to know what happened or her work colleagues.

Krista is not taking any contraception at the moment, she only uses condoms. I explain how the morning-after pill works and that if she has any doubts, she should do a pregnancy test if her period is late. No form of contraception is 100%. Now, I advise her of the contraceptive options open to her including the longer-lasting ones like the implant and the coil and advise her to book an appointment with the nurse to get a more reliable form of contraception. After printing off the prescription and informing her the prescription is ready, I finish the call and add an information leaflet about the long-acting reversible forms of contraception to the prescription.

* * *

The second ring-back is from the mum of an eight-month-old baby with a temperature. William has been coughing for the last day and although mum is not excessively concerned about him, she would still prefer to have him checked over today.

Rather than phoning mum, I send a task to the receptionists to offer mum a sit-and-wait appointment at ten past ten for William. This is followed by the advice to contact us again if she becomes more concerned about him or if she is very concerned to ring 999. It is important to cover all possibilities.

Sit-and-wait appointments are non-existent appointments. I make them up as I go along. The timing is a rough estimate of when the patient will be seen and as the name states; the patient comes in and tells the receptionist he or she has arrived, then takes a seat and waits until I can see them.

Two ring-backs down, another four to go. Unless more have arrived in the meantime, of course.

* * *

The third ring-back is from twenty-two-year-old Sam, who has suffered from a sore throat since this morning. Sam is otherwise well and wants to be seen and have antibiotics for his throat. Really? A sore throat since that morning is urgent?

As it is very unlikely his problem is urgent, I decide to leave it for now and return to this ring-back later. I will first check the other ring-backs.

* * *

The fourth ring-back is from eighty-five-year-old Brian, who suffers from a painful right knee since yesterday. Brian has not injured it, but it is swollen and painful.

Again I sent a task to the receptionists to invite him for a sit-and-wait appointment, this time at twenty past ten. I wonder if he has an attack of gout.

* * *

The fifth ring-back is from thirty-five-year-old Melanie, who has been trying to book an appointment for the last week without any success. She has tried to phone every day her notes state.

Really? As I turn my thoughts to last week, I distinctly

remember noticing unbooked appointments every day last week, even as late as four in the afternoon appointments remained available. Last week was a rather unusual week as we tend to be overbooked. No, it is far more likely that the appointments offered to Melanie last week were not to her liking. Either the appointments offered were with a doctor she didn't wish to see or they were at a time that didn't suit Melanie. It is even possible she did not try to ring at all, but is just playing on the usual lack of appointments to put more pressure on us to provide her with one.

Melanie has told the receptionist she has taken this morning off especially to get an appointment and now no appointments are left for today, which is unacceptable. She needs to be seen today and feels her problem is urgent. Melanie suffers from hair loss.

Although Melanie's problem may seem urgent to her, it is not medically urgent. For the moment, I will leave this problem and come back to it later.

* * *

Already I'm looking at the sixth ring-back. By now it is twenty-seven minutes past eight and the first patient has arrived. Still, I decide to action one more ring-back before calling the first patient in. It promises to be a busy morning already.

Amy is a three-year-old girl, whose mum phoned as she has a temperature. Amy complains of an earache and has been crying all night. After mum gave her some paracetamol at half-past seven, she appears to be more settled and has even fallen asleep. Mum does not consider her to be seriously ill, but wonders if she has an ear infection and would like her to be seen.

Another task makes its way to the receptionists to invite Amy for a half-past ten sit-and-wait appointment.

Now it is time to start the normal surgery.

CHAPTER 7

Tuesday, 8:29 am

At twenty-nine minutes past eight, I press the button to call in the first patient. This will sound a buzzer in reception and the receptionist will send in my patient. While I wait for fifty-six-year-old Stuart to come in, I check the last few entries on his notes. He consulted a locum about two weeks ago with symptoms of heartburn and indigestion. The locum diagnosed him with acid reflux and started him on medication for this and Stuart was advised to return for a review of his symptoms after two weeks. This is likely why Stuart has come today.

There is a knock on the door, "Come in."

Stuart enters, "Morning, doc."

I offer Stuart a seat and ask what I can do for him today.

"Well, I saw this locum bloke two weeks ago for my acid and he gave me these lansoppy things and asked me to come back after two weeks to let you know how I was getting on with them."

"And, how have you been getting on with the lansoprazole?"

Stuart tells me his symptoms have nearly completely left him and he is very happy with them. He has experienced no side-effects.

When I check some basic background information, Stuart confirms he still smokes twenty-five cigarettes a day, drinks three cans of lager at night and loves spicy food. He is also overweight.

After informing him that acid reflux tends to be worse in people with a history like his and that stopping smoking, reducing his alcohol intake and avoiding spicy food may help to improve his symptoms, not to mention the positive effect weight loss will have on his symptoms, Stuart appears to feel happy he can do something to control his symptoms himself. Prescription charges are considerable after all and if he can avoid those, he will be much happier.

"I would advise you to continue with the medication for the moment until the pack is finished. You can try without them at that point, but if your symptoms recur or worsen, you need to see us again."

Stuart leaves with a smile on his face, he is adamant to try the changes in lifestyle and improve his symptoms.

* * *

After Stuart leaves, I enter the details and advice I gave him on Stuart's medical notes and check the appointment screen. The next patient has not arrived yet, but another two ring-backs have appeared on the screen and I check those while waiting for the next patient to arrive. There is no point wasting a single minute if the day is likely to be busy.

* * *

The seventh ring-back of this morning is from fifty-two-year-old Lucy, who, the receptionist noted on the records, sounded distressed on the phone and was in tears. Lucy informed Michelle that she was crying all the time since her mum passed away two days ago. She denied any suicidal thoughts.

Thanks, Michelle for checking that out already. Michelle is a very experienced receptionist who already knows what questions we likely want an answer to.

Now, I send a task to the receptionists to invite Lucy for a twenty to eleven sit-and-wait appointment and book it in as a twenty-minute appointment. A patient in distress will need extra time, the normal ten-minute appointment will not suffice.

* * *

Now I turn my attention to the eighth ring-back, five-year-old Eli, who has suffered from a rash for the last five weeks, which is not improving. The rash has not changed and Eli is otherwise well. Mum is worried he has meningitis and wants him checked over.

My thoughts do not mirror mum's worries. Several things point to this being something different from meningitis. Meningitis leaves the patient extremely unwell, the rash is of a much shorter duration, hours rather than weeks.

I send a task to the receptionist to offer another sit-and-wait appointment, this one for eleven and add the advice to contact us again if Eli's condition worsens and if he gets very poorly, she should ring 999 instead. This advice feels unnecessary at the moment, but it is important to cover all bases.

* * *

By now the second patient has arrived. After I press the buzzer, I check thirty-seven-year-old Ryan's notes while I wait for him to arrive. Ryan is a known patient who has seen us regularly over the last four months with depression and anxiety. For the last three months, he has been given sick notes as he was unable to cope at work. He is not suicidal and is seeing the Psychological Wellbeing Practitioner (PWP for short) for counselling.

Today Ryan tells me he is feeling much better and although he is not quite ready to go back to work yet, he hopes to be ready for work in two weeks.

"Can I have another note for two weeks, please, doctor? I hope I will be able to go back to work after that." A hopeful expression rests on his face.

As I hand him the note, I notice how his eye contact has improved significantly over the last few weeks and today he has shaved as well after having appeared to be rather unkempt over recent months.

Yes, hopefully, he will soon be fit for work again.

* * *

When Ryan leaves a few minutes later it is a quarter to nine. The next patient is due at ten to nine and has not arrived yet. This gives me a chance to check on any ring-backs that may have arrived again.

And yes, as was to be expected, another three ring-backs arrived already. I also notice there are thirty-seven electronic prescriptions waiting and I quickly go to the prescription screen and sign those. I like having zeroes in the bottom row whenever possible to tell me there is nothing waiting. Unfortunately, that does not often happen in real life. At least, not for long.

* * *

Ring-back number nine is from fifty-five-year-old Lesley. She requests an urgent issue of her repeat prescriptions. She has run out of the medication over the weekend - hang on it's Tuesday today, why does she contact us now? - and wants us to do an urgent prescription. Lesley apologised for the inconvenience, she forgot to put her repeat prescription in on time.

Will people ever learn? The rules are that once a patient hands in a repeat prescription request, we have forty-eight hours during working days to fill that request. For the non-repeat items they request a repeat prescription of, patients should allow a week for this to be processed.

First, I check what medication Lesley is on and none of these are essential for her health. She has painkillers on the list and Gaviscon. As I am already looking at the repeat list, it is easier to just issue and print, although this does not follow our own rules. After the signing the prescription, I put it to the side to take to reception later on, then send a task to the receptionists to inform the patient to pick up the prescription tonight and add a little reminder to the prescription to request prescriptions on time in future.

* * *

The tenth ring-back is for information only.

Elaine spoke to the wife of fifty-two-year-old Jonathan. He is complaining of pain centrally on the chest which takes his breath away and he is sweaty and clammy. Elaine has already advised them to ring 999 and the wife will do this.

I add a message to the notes to state I agree with the action Elaine has taken and sent her a message to compliment her on her action and thank her for it.

Jonathan may have a heart attack and time is of the essence. Any delay could decrease his chances of survival or of a good quality of life afterwards.

* * *

My next patient hasn't arrived yet. Another two minutes until his appointment is due. I use this time to check the eleventh ring-back. Mum phoned about ten-year-old Olivia who has suffered from diarrhoea and vomiting since this morning. She would like some advice.

As I pick up the phone, I ring mum back. When I ask what the problem is, I already know some of it but always like to hear it again in mum's own words, mum tells me that Olivia woke up with a tummy ache around five this morning. She came over to see mum to let her know and then was violently sick on the floor beside mum's bed.

The disgust can be discovered clearly in mum's voice as she remembers. Yes, the joys of motherhood include cleaning up after your poorly kids.

Olivia has not been sick since, but she has had diarrhoea twice since six this morning. Although she has a slight tummy ache, Olivia appears to be otherwise well, mum says. When I ask whether she has a temperature or any urinary symptoms, mum denies this.

In the background I can make out Olivia calling, "Mum, can I have some toast? I'm hungry."

"No, you can't have anything while you are ill, I already told you so earlier."

"But mu-um."

Mum then speaks to me again and asks for confirmation she is doing the right thing by denying Olivia food.

Instead, I tell her that if Olivia feels like eating, she is allowed to eat. If it makes her symptoms worse, she can always cut down on it then. The most important thing is to make sure Olivia does not get dehydrated, so I advise mum to give her plenty of fluids if she can tolerate them and to also drink some soup or stock to replenish the salts she loses by being sick and having the runs.

After advising mum to get back in touch if Olivia does not improve or if she gets worse, I finish the call.

* * *

By now it is seven to nine and the next patient has arrived. Melissa is a forty-five-year-old lady, who complains of urinary incontinence, or accidents as she calls them, when she coughs, sneezes or laughs. She has no problems losing control of her bladder when she feels the need to go to the toilet. Melissa tells me this has been ongoing for the last year, but so far she has been too embarrassed to consult the doctor about it, instead suffering in silence. She has also waited to see me as she prefers to consult a woman for this problem.

Her problem appears to be what we call stress incontinence, with symptoms exactly like the ones described above.

Melissa agrees to an internal examination and soon I confirm she suffers from a slight prolapse, the bladder wall hangs down in the vagina a little lower than it should do. This is a very common problem and often due to weak pelvic floor muscles. Sometimes the patient can remedy this herself by doing frequent pelvic floor exercises.

These are done by squeezing the muscles in the area,

the usual recommendation is to do twelve fast ones, followed by twelve slow ones, holding the muscle tensed for twelve seconds if possible, followed by another twelve fast ones. This should be done every hour, on the hour, of the waking hours.

 In reality, this is unlikely to happen. Women lead busy lives and will forget to do their exercises as a result.

 I give her the advice and ask her to return in a month to let me know if there is any improvement in her symptoms.

* * *

 After Melissa has left, I notice another ring-back has arrived. I take a quick look and decide this one will have to wait. By now it is three minutes past nine and my fourth patient is waiting.

 Twenty-three-year-old Chelsea is five months pregnant and has come to see me with a cough she has had for the last week. She is a known asthmatic and has needed to use her blue inhaler a bit more frequent. Chelsea tells me she has been bringing up green phlegm and has run a bit of a temperature. She is unsure how high as she has not got a thermometer at home.

 When I listen to her lungs, there are some crackles present on the right, confirming a chest infection.

Unfortunately, Chelsea is allergic to penicillin and we have to choose an alternative antibiotic which is safe for her and the baby.

After advising Chelsea to seek medical attention if her symptoms don't improve or if they worsen, she leaves.

* * *

My fifth patient of the day turns out to be a difficult and emotional one. Forty-seven-year-old Moira comes in and after asking what I can do for her today, Moira collapses in floods of tears, "Oh doctor, I'm so depressed. I have been suffering from depression all my life, or at least it seems that way, and everything is just not getting any better. At times I think I would be better off if I was not here. But then I remember the children and pull myself together again as best I can."

When I ask Moira if she considers she could ever act on those feelings, Moira denies that, "Oh no, I could never do that, no way," and Moira shakes her head, "Barry has told me I really need to see you again," Moira looks down to the hands she has folded in her lap, "I can't stand it when Barry touches me and I think he has finally had enough. Who would want someone who doesn't want to be touched?" More tears roll down Moira's face and I grab a box of tissues and place the box on the desk in case Moira needs the tissues.

"Is there anything that has caused you to feel this way?"

Moira seems to consider this for a moment, "Well, uh..., I have never told this to anyone, but when I was twelve our next-door neighbour raped me. Although I tried to avoid Nick ever since, he would often babysit us when our parents went for a night out. Every time he looked after us, Nick would sneak into my bedroom at night and rape me again. At the time, I was too scared to tell my parents about this, Nick said he would kill them if I did, and I never told anyone about it."

Tears continue to roll down Moira's face as my heart squeezes painfully. I find it difficult to breathe and all my willpower focuses on remaining in control and not showing my emotions, "You have told no one about this?"

Moira shakes her head, "No, you are the first person I've ever told about this. The worst thing is, Nick still lives only a street away from us and I run into him on a regular basis. But I just can't cope with this any longer."

She looks down for a moment, "When I was pregnant with the kids I was terrified. Fortunately, both are boys, thank God. I wouldn't have known what to do if the kids were girls. How could I protect them?"

We discuss the local rape and sexual abuse counselling service where Moira can self-refer to and I offer my support. Has Moira considered reporting Nick to the police? If not for herself then to perhaps stop this from happening to others? Moira has considered this, but so far seemed uncertain and worried that she might not be believed. She does not feel he still poses a risk to others, he had a massive stroke a few years ago, is wheelchair bound and unable to do much for himself, let alone to others.

When she leaves she looks much happier, now realising it was not her fault this happened to her, although still not really believing it.

"Can I hug you doctor?"

She hugs me before leaving and asks if she can come to talk to me again. Of course she can. Even if it is emotionally draining, I'm happy to speak to her again if she feels the need. I only advise her to make a double appointment if she does. This appointment has taken twenty-five minutes after all and I'm now running behind.

* * *

After Moira leaves, I spot another three ring-backs arrived. I'm running more than a quarter of an hour behind and I need to catch up. The receptionists would alert me if anything urgent had popped up and I leave the ring-backs for now and buzz for the next patient instead of checking the ring-backs.

Immediately an instant message pops up on the screen from Elaine, "Be careful with this patient, Dr Ellen. He was very agitated and verbally aggressive in the waiting area."

Forty-three-year-old Darren blazes in without knocking, his face like thunder, "This is absolutely ridiculous. Do you think I have all the time in the world? For me, time is money. If I take time off to see the doctor, I don't get paid and I expect to be seen on time. The service you provide here is completely atrocious. This is unacceptable and I should go to my member of parliament over this." Darren's demeanour is such that images of cartoon characters with steam coming out of their ears come to mind.

No 'hello' or even giving me a chance to apologise first. No, Darren steamrolls his way into my room and airs his anger. He remained standing while he spoke, his posture aggressive and looming over me, an attempt to intimidate me further. Now he sits down, sliding down on the chair, his face still like thunder.

How can I save the situation? "I'm genuinely sorry to keep you waiting. You are absolutely right that it is unacceptable to keep you waiting for such a long time and I take full responsibility for that. I apologise sincerely." I take a breath, "So what can I do for you today?" and hope my apology will calm him down a bit, the fact I agree it is unacceptable may take the wind from his sails.

"Well, I don't really have the time for this, but now I'm here," he takes out a piece of paper with writing on it. "First of all, I have an ingrowing toenail and want some antibiotics for that. Second, I have this nasty cough for the last week and need antibiotics to clear that. And the third problem is this rash on my leg that has been bothering me for a few weeks. It's itchy and you need to do something about that."

How should I respond to this? At the surgery, we maintain a simple rule, One appointment, One patient, One problem. Instead, Darren expects me to deal with three problems at the same time and I am already running late. Every problem deserves their own proper attention and trying to force three problems within one appointment may make this difficult.

I try to explain to Darren that we usually only allow one problem per appointment to allow it to get the attention it deserves, but I notice how he only gets more agitated and instead inform him we will explore his problems today.

When I check his toenail, the nail is indeed growing in slightly, but it is not infected and does not require any treatment at the moment, "Daily bathing of the toe will help to avoid this getting infected. Just ten minutes in warm water and soaking it before dabbing it dry. If the toe does get infected after all, then please come back to have it checked."

Darren sits up a little straighter, "Well that's a bloody waste of time. I need you to give me some antibiotics for this now and make the wait worth my time. I haven't got time to come back if it gets worse, I need this sorting out now."

Next, we turn our attention to his cough. Darren doesn't cough up any phlegm and has no temperature. His chest is clear on examination. Again there is no reason to prescribe antibiotics and this would be bad practice.

"You're bloody no good. You call yourself a doctor?" Darren sits up even straighter and leans forward a little.

Darren's last problem is the itchy rash on his leg. So far, he has not tried anything for it, instead he wants me to sort the problem for him. On examination there is mild eczema and I advise him to use a moisturiser for it. When I offer to write a prescription, Darren refuses and leans forward more, invading my personal space as he does, "You're a bloody disgrace, you've kept me waiting for half an hour and have done nothing for me." Darren stands up and struts out of the room, slamming the door behind him.

I let out a deep breath of relief and wonder how I could have handled that better. Hopefully, his rants are sufficient for him, but I fear more is to follow. Is this job even worth it?

Darren's behaviour has also allowed my insecurities to resurge. Will I ever be good enough? Is he correct and am I disgrace? Should I just give up and admit I will never measure up to his standards or those of my dad?

Still, I won't let this beat me and pull up my big girl panties to continue with the next patient on my list.

* * *

Following Darren's outburst, I'm running behind even more. By now, It is nine minutes to ten and the next patient was due at half-past nine. I notice even more ring-backs arrived, but they will need to wait until I have finished morning surgery.

Libby is a three-year-old girl who comes with her mum. When she enters she runs straight over and holds out her hands to ask me to lift her up. Libby climbs on my lap and hugs me. If Libby was not someone who would come to see us regularly, this would be a worrying sign, raising concerns about possible child abuse. Libby, however, is a regular, and she loves to cuddle. The little hug she gives me makes up for the difficult consultation I had before and makes me feel like this job is worth it after all.

"Look, I've got a poorly," Libby holds out her right index finger. She has bitten her nails, and it is a little bit red around the nailbed. Not quite infected, but mum will need to keep an eye on it.

When I open my mouth to advise mum of this, the phone rings, "I'm sorry, I have to take this, I'm on call today."

Mum nods.

"Sorry to disturb you, Dr Ellen. The district nurse would like to have a word with you. She is with the patient now."

Libby puts the call through and the district nurse tells me about the patient she is with. He is an eighty-seven-year-old gentleman with an oozing wound on his leg with redness and a slight discharge. Does she need to do swabs or will I start antibiotics without them? The district nurse does not consider it is bad enough for antibiotics at the moment and will visit the patient again in two days. I advise her to take swabs and unless it deteriorates, we will wait for the results of the swabs before starting antibiotics.

After putting down the phone, I turn to mum, "Now where were we?" Next, I advise bathing the poorly finger and to return if the symptoms don't improve or worsen. I also tell Libby to not bite her lips and she solemnly nods her head in agreement.

* * *

I'm still running fifteen minutes behind. By now my bladder is bursting, but I first want to finish seeing the patients waiting for me.

Seventeen-year-old Abigail has come for a pill check. She is on one of the combined pills and it suits her well and Abigail wishes to continue with it. Further questioning reveals she does not smoke, and on examining her, Abigail has a normal weight and her blood pressure is normal. Abigail has no history of medical conditions making the pill a safe option for her and she is not keen on trying any of the long-acting forms of contraception. After checking she still knows what to do if she forgets a pill and is aware that antibiotics, vomiting and diarrhoea may interfere with the effectiveness of the pill, she leaves.

Eight patients seen, one more to go. That is before seeing the extras and responding to the ring-backs.

* * *

Unfortunately, I have not yet managed to catch up. I'm still running fifteen minutes behind. At six minutes past ten, it is unlikely I will start with the extra patients at the time I had hoped to.

Fifty-four-year-old Heather is on hormone replacement therapy (HRT) for menopausal symptoms. Heather has been using this for two years and feels happy with it. Her blood pressure is normal, she is up to date with her smears and checks her breasts regularly. Heather's last mammogram was last year. Again we double check she has no contraindications for continued use of HRT, then agree to review again in a year. Before Heather leaves, I remind her HRT is recommended to be used for a maximum of five years.

* * *

At last, the last booked patient has been seen and I get up to use the bathroom. First, I pick up the prescriptions I have done during the surgery and take them to reception. Although I am very aware there are patients waiting for me already, I desperately need to use the bathroom.

My face feels hot as the pressure of work weighs down on me. Still, I will need to remain in control. If I don't, then who will? When I check my face in the mirror, it is bright red. I throw some water in my face in an attempt to cool down, then dab it dry and leave the bathroom again.

When I return to my room, I quickly check the list of ring-backs received. A receptionist has placed several 'urgent prescriptions' on my desk waiting to be signed. I really need to speak to Patricia about what is and what isn't an urgent prescription. Maybe she has forgotten we have a list of medications that need to be issued as a priority as the patient's life relies on them.

CHAPTER 8

Tuesday, 10:20 am

When I return to my room after the brief bathroom break, I find fifteen ring-backs waiting for me on top of the patients I offered sit-and-wait appointments. I quickly check some ring-backs.

Ring-back number twelve was a mum who phoned about her seven-year-old daughter Emma, who has a tummy ache and this is worsening. I send a task to the receptionist to invite Emma for a sit-and-wait appointment and twenty past eleven and ask her to bring a urine sample to the appointment.

The thirteenth ring-back is from fifty-two-year old Michelle, who suffers from urinary symptoms and suspects she has a urine infection. Michelle wants to be seen to have this confirmed and treated. Instead, I sent another task and ask the receptionists to ask Michelle to bring in a urine sample, we can deal with the problem on the basis of that, avoiding unnecessary waits for Michelle and unnecessary appointments for us. At reception, we have a form the patient has to fill in when handing in a urine sample. First is this for a suspected infection or for a pregnancy test, name, address and date of birth are also required and symptoms the patient has. It also asks about whether the patient is pregnant or has any allergies to medication. Although these details should in principle also be on the patient's notes, it never hurts to double-check.

The fourteenth ring-back is from the district nurse. She is requesting a visit for eighty-six-year-old Bill, who she suspects has a chest infection. She feels he needs to be seen. When I look at Bill's notes, I notice he has attended with his daughter a month ago. I sent a task to the receptionists to check if Bill is able to get to the surgery and if so, I will see him around half-past eleven. If this is not possible, I will have to visit around lunchtime instead.

The pressure is building and heat rises further in my face, my head pounds and my heart seems to want to leave my chest. And it is only twenty past ten. Most of the day still lies ahead and with it the expectation of more ring-backs and emergencies.

* * *

Before seeing the first extra patient, I decide to phone the third ring-back for that morning.

Twenty-two-year-old Sam phoned this morning about his sore throat. As I do not expect this to be anything serious, I hope I can solve this over the phone. The sore throat has only been present since this morning after all.

"Hello?"

After confirming I'm speaking to Sam, he tells me his throat has now improved and no longer giving any problems. After giving Sam some supportive advice to help with a sore throat and telling him to seek medical attention if his throat would worsen again, we end the call. He is happy to find out he could also see the minor illness nurse or even a pharmacist with these symptoms if needed.

* * *

The first extra patient is eight-month-old William, the second ring-back of the day. The first things I notice when William and his mum enter the room are his watery eyes and snotty nose. And, of course, the massive smile on William's face. The cough is still present and his temperature is a little raised at 37.8 degrees Celsius. Mum tells me she has last given him paracetamol four hours before.

I check William over. Throat normal, some small glands in his neck, his right eardrum is red and his chest is clear. He has no known allergies and I give mum a prescription for amoxicillin to treat his ear infection, advising mum to return if his symptoms don't improve or if they worsen.

* * *

Now It is time for eighty-five-year-old Brian to come in. He was the fourth ring-back and scheduled for twenty past ten, but it is already twenty to eleven instead.

"It's my knee, doc. I think it may be gout."

When I ask Brian why he thinks it is, he informs me he has suffered from gout for a few years and this feels exactly like it did before.

On examination, his right knee is swollen, red and hot to the touch. Next, I double check his notes and he indeed was diagnosed with gout previously, which was also confirmed with a blood test. Brian receives no medication for his gout at the moment and I give him some painkillers to help him with the pain and swelling.

"Once the gout has fully settled, it may be worth to consider giving you something to lower the uric acid in your blood. This may help to prevent you from having these attacks so often."

"Why can't you give me that medication now, doc?"

Now I need to explain how the medication that helps to reduce the risk of having further attacks actually worsens the acute attack and that we, therefore, need to wait until the current attack has finished. Brian is happy with the explanation and leaves with the prescription for pain relief.

* * *

The third patient booked as an extra is the sixth ring-back of this morning. Three-year-old Amy attends with her grandma, "Sorry, Amy's mum had to go to work. I'm Amy's grandma."

With a snotty nose and watery eyes, the cold symptoms are obvious. Amy's temperature is normal at 37.3, her throat and chest are clear and she has a few small glands in her neck. Amy's left eardrum is red, however, and I give her a prescription for an antibiotic, erythromycin once we discover from her notes and grandma that Amy is allergic to penicillin. A pity, most children hate the taste of it.

While I'm in the middle of explaining the findings and treatment to Amy's grandma, an instant message pops up from the practice manager, "Can you see me when you have a minute, please?"

That is never good news. With the realisation how busy the morning is already, I sent a quick message back to inform her it is rather busy at the moment, but I will try after surgery.

I continue the explanations and advice to grandma and Amy soon leaves. My stress levels have reached another high.

* * *

Still, I battle on and call the next extra patient in. It is fifty-two-year-old Lucy, the distressed lady who lost her mum two days ago. After offering my condolences for her loss, I allow Lucy to tell me her story.

Sobbing and with red-rimmed eyes, Lucy starts to talk. She has no makeup on, her hair is uncombed and she wipes her nose with a crumpled tissue. Lucy continues to play with the tissue the entire consultation, makes little to no eye contact and cries incessantly.

"It is not fair. Mum was such a lovely lady. And to think she died like that. It's just not fair."

Lucy's mum was diagnosed with ovarian cancer three months ago. Mum had no symptoms of the disease until it was too late and only consulted her GP when she appeared to be six months pregnant. Something not possible for an eighty-four-year-old. The diagnosis was a shock to the entire family, but especially to Lucy, who had a very close relationship with her mum, "Why did she leave me? How could she do that to me? She knew I needed her."

Lucy also wonders why the illness was not discovered earlier and was angry with the GP involved. From what I understood from Lucy, her mum had not seen the doctor in years until about three and a half months ago and a diagnosis had followed fairly soon after.

Supporting and soothing Lucy as much as possible, I offer her further support, hand her a leaflet to tell her about the grief process to reassure her the feelings she is battling through are normal for the situation. I also offer to see her again for a review, which she gratefully accepts.

Lucy's eyes are still red, but she looks less distressed than she did on arrival.

* * *

The fifth extra patient was booked for eleven as a sit-and-wait. At the moment, I'm running twenty minutes behind schedule and although I consider this to be not bad going after the morning I have had so far, I still don't like it.

Five-year-old Eli enters with his mum. He is the little boy who has had a rash for five weeks and mum is concerned this would be meningitis. Eli skips in the room and runs around, playing aeroplane.

As soon as mum enters the room she starts a tirade, "How could you keep him waiting? I was told to get here for eleven and it is already twenty past. Eli could have died in that time!" Mum's face is crimson and spittle leaves her mouth with every spoken word. Her eyes are wide open and she appears panicked.

Yes, as though I simply sat here, twiddling my thumbs. Instead of showing my feelings, I take a breath, "I'm really sorry to keep you waiting. You are absolutely right to be angry about that. Did the receptionist not mention this was a sit-and-wait appointment?"

There is no doubt in my mind she will have informed mum of this, they are very meticulous in informing patients that the time is merely an indication and that the doctor will see them when able to do so.

Mum nods her head and relaxes a little, "I'm sorry, I've just been so worried. He has had this rash for a while and it's not getting any better."

Then I suggest we look at the rash while asking how long Eli has had the rash for and how he is in himself.

The rash has been present for five weeks; it seems to get worse, and it is itchy. Eli has been fine in himself the entire time. Examination shows the rash to be eczema and I explain this to mum, offering a prescription for a cream to help Eli with this.

While I print off the prescription, an instant message pops up from Deborah, our nurse, "Can you pop in for a moment in between patients?" and I reply I will.

* * *

When Eli leaves, I pick up a few prescriptions I signed in between patients and take them to reception, and rush to the nurse's room.

Deborah has a patient with her for a change of a ring pessary and she wants my opinion on whether to replace the ring or leave it out for a while. She has noticed that the patient's vagina is rather red and sore looking and wonders if it is perhaps better to let it heal a little first.

After checking the irritated area myself, I agree with Deborah and advise the patient to return in two weeks for another attempt. Hopefully, the area will have healed enough by then.

* * *

Now it is time to go back to my room for the next emergency patient. Seven-year-old Emma attends with her mum. She started with a tummy ache in her lower abdomen yesterday evening, initially around her bellybutton, but this has now moved to the right lower tummy. The pain has gradually become worse, and she has had a small amount of diarrhoea, but not passed any further 'number twos' since last night. Emma denies any urinary symptoms and when I check the urine she has brought, it is indeed clear.

"So, how did you come to the surgery this morning?"

Mum looks confused, "We drove here."

I turn to Emma and ask her if she had any pain while mum drove here and she mentions the pain was worse when they drove over speed bumps. At my request, Emma jumps up on the couch and I examine her tummy. There is an obvious tenderness on the right-hand side and I suspect she has appendicitis. It is time to inform Emma and mum and phone the hospital to request admission for their opinion.

When I phone the hospital it takes a moment before switchboard answers. They put me through and again I have to wait for someone to answer the phone. After I explain the symptoms and the findings they accept the referral and I hang up.

While explaining the directions given by the hospital, I write a referral letter and hand it to mum to take to the hospital with her.

"Mum, can I have my crisps now? You promised."

Uh, no, that is not such a good idea. I explain that until we know if my suspicion is correct and whether surgery is needed, it is best not to eat or drink anything. Mum nods and after wishing them luck, they leave.

The emergency referral has brought along another delay, and it is now ten to twelve.

* * *

Now it is the turn for eighty-six-year-old Bill to be seen. He was the gentleman the district nurse requested a visit for, but fortunately, his daughter was able to bring him to the surgery instead. Bill is known with COPD, also known as chronic bronchitis. He used to be a miner in the past and was a smoker until fifteen years ago. His breathing has been worse over the last few days, he is coughing up green phlegm and sounds wheezy on arrival.

When I check his chest, there are crackles on the left side. Bill's temperature appears to be fine at 37.5 and his oxygen levels are okay at 92%. These are his usual levels. With the chest infection confirmed, I issue him a prescription for antibiotics, a look at his notes alerting me he needs a two-week course rather than a one week course as he is known with bronchiectasis.

It is always difficult to explain to a patient what this means. Basically, the lungs are not just large empty bags. Instead, they are full of tiny little round spaces, a bit like grapes on a vine. In the case of bronchiectasis, some of these little areas have burst and become a larger area with the surrounding round spaces. This means there is less lung tissue to absorb the oxygen in the air from, but it also leaves larger pockets which can easily become infected. And if they become infected, it takes longer than one week of antibiotics to get rid of this.

The usual advice to seek medical attention if no better or worse follows and Bill and his daughter leave.

* * *

For a moment, I sit back in my chair and rub my neck. It is aching and my head throbs. Still, more work is waiting for me and I need to get back to it. There is no time to take a minute and relax; patients are waiting to be seen.

I take an instant to go through the remaining ring-backs.

The lady with the hair loss is still waiting to hear back from me. This is, however, non-urgent and I will try to fit her in if I can. It is twelve already and my stomach is protesting. No time for the wicked though and my stomach will have to wait. Instead, I pour another cup of tea.

The urine sample I requested for the fifty-two-year-old lady with a possible urine infection is still awaited. I can't finalise that one yet.

The fifteenth ring-back is, however, a urine sample for a different patient with a possible urine infection. As the sample was clear, I send a task to the receptionists to inform the patient of this.

The next nine ring-backs are prescription requests from the district nurse, nursing homes and patients and a urine sample and they can wait till later.

There are two visit requests from a nursing home and I will look at those in a minute and I turn my attention to the twenty-seventh patient on the ring-back list.

This is twenty-seven-year-old Joshua, who is known with asthma and has been suffering from a cough for five days. He is bringing up green phlegm, his chest feels tight and he would like to be seen. I send a task to the receptionists to offer him a sit-and-wait appointment for half-past twelve.

Ring-back number twenty-eight is from forty-seven-year-old David, who thinks he has conjunctivitis. Although this could also be seen and treated by the pharmacist, I send a task to invite him for a sit-and-wait appointment at twenty to one.

Next, I check the prescription requests and urine samples while waiting for the next emergency appointments to arrive.

* * *

The first request is from the district nurse for dressings for a housebound patient with leg ulcers. The request is simple and I issue the prescription and sign this before adding it to the pile with signed prescriptions. A task to the receptionists to inform the patient the prescription is ready for collection and it is time to move on to the seventeenth ring-back on the list.

* * *

The next one is another request for dressings from the district nurse. With difficulty I find the ones she has requested, I issue and print the prescription and after signing add it to the growing pile. Another task is sent and I move on to the eighteenth ring-back.

* * *

The third prescription request is a request for catheter bags and equipment. This takes five minutes before I am able to find the exact ones the district nurse has requested, I issue, print and sign the prescription and send another task off to inform the receptionists.

* * *

A little variation. The nineteenth ring-back on the list is a urine sample result. A forty-four-year-old lady has brought in a sample for a suspected urine infection. She is not pregnant, and the sample is suggestive of infection. As far as I can tell from her notes, this is the first infection she has suffered with and I issue a prescription, taking note of the fact she has no known allergies.

Once the prescription is ready, I send a task to the receptionists to inform the patient of the results and that the prescription is ready for collection. I also advise to seek medical attention if the symptoms do not improve after a few days or if they worsen and to see a doctor if she suffers any further urine infections.

And it is time to move on to the twentieth ring-back on the list.

* * *

This ring-back is a prescription request from one of our COPD patients. Samuel has a self-management plan and as part of that has been advised to always keep a supply of antibiotics ready for infections. Samuel knows how to use the colour chart to determine if his sputum is suggestive of infection and at which time to start on his antibiotics. If the course of antibiotics would not improve his symptoms or clear the infection, he is aware he should see the doctor, but otherwise, Samuel phones for another supply to have on hand for the next time he requires them.

Samuel started taking antibiotics yesterday and is already feeling a little better. Next, I check when he last received a supply, which was six months ago and issue the prescription. He is a sensible man.

* * *

The next ring-back is a request for aqueous cream for a nursing home patient and after I issue the requested prescription, I send a task to the receptionists to inform the home the prescription is ready for collection.

* * *

The same nursing home requests dressings for a resident with leg ulcers, and again I issue a prescription and send a task to the girls. This is a repeat of a prescription given at an earlier time and only takes a few minutes.

* * *

The twenty-third ring-back is another prescription request from another nursing home. This time for lactulose for a patient with constipation. Lactulose is on their home remedies list and if it helps; they ask for a prescription from the doctor. Another task to the receptionist after I issue the prescription.

* * *

The twenty-fourth ring-back is slightly trickier. A nursing home has received a new resident and they request a prescription of the patient's repeat medication for three days, to bring this in line with the medications for the other residents. To do this, I need to issue all the repeat medications, then go back into them and adjust the duration times to three days. With the list this patient has, it takes ten minutes. When I have completed it, I send another task to the receptionists to inform them.

* * *

Next on the list are the requests from another nursing home. The twenty-fifth ring-back is a request for five days worth of medications to bring them in line with the other residents and I sort that and send a task to inform the receptionists this is completed.

While looking through the ring-back list I have already noticed two visit requests from the same nursing home. Although I am on my own now, I still decide they need to be looked at today.

The thirty-third ring-back was a request to visit eighty-nine-year-old Joseph at the nursing home. He is coughing and they wonder if he suffers from a chest infection.

The next visit request is for 101-year-old Muriel, who has a skin lesion on her forehead and they would like an opinion on that while I see Joseph, anyway.

I send a task to the receptionists for both patients, to confirm I will attempt to visit both patients around lunchtime.

* * *

The next ring-back on the list is a request from the district nurse. Seventy-three-year-old Thomas is a terminally ill patient with lung cancer. His pain is such that he currently has a syringe driver. This means that he has a constant infusion of pain relief under the skin, often together with medications to stop nausea, excess secretions and panic. The instructions are only valid for five days and a new instruction then needs to be written. Even if there are no changes to the dosages, another one is needed and today that task falls to me.

After carefully double checking the previous instructions and the notes left on the notes by the district nurses, I complete a new version of the instruction. This is now ready to be faxed to the district nurse. As I prefer to do nearly everything electronic, I have already completed the form on the notes of the patient and then printed it off. It saves the file room clerk the job of scanning the form onto the notes and it also ensures the form is legible.

I send a task to inform the receptionists and move on to the next job.

* * *

Twenty-seven-year-old Joshua is next, the asthmatic with a possible chest infection. When he hobbles in, I notice the wheezing and as I check his chest there are obvious crackles on the left side of his chest. His oxygen levels are good at 98%, and his peakflow, another measurement to check his breathlessness, is 470, which is acceptable for Joshua. After checking he still has a supply of his inhalers and issuing a prescription for antibiotics, Joshua leaves with the advice to seek medical attention if his symptoms don't improve or worsen.

* * *

Nearly a quarter to one and I'm finally starting to see the light at the end of the tunnel. My next patient is forty-seven-year-old David who believes he has conjunctivitis. His left eye is a little watery and looks slightly pink, but there is no sign of a bacterial form of conjunctivitis. The eye is itchy, but he does not experience any pain in the eye or problems tolerating the light. When I check his glands, there are a few palpable in front of his left ear. This also suggests his conjunctivitis is viral rather than bacterial.

With advice to wash out the eyes with cooled down, boiled water and to review if the problem worsens, adding this could be seen by the minor illness nurse or the pharmacist, David leaves.

* * *

By now the urine sample for the fifty-two-year-old lady from the thirteenth ring-back has finally been received. The sample indeed shows signs of infection. As she has no known allergies, and no previous urine infections I can find on her notes nor any medication preventing the use of certain antibiotics, I issue the prescription, in view of the fact she is generally unwell with the urinary symptoms, and send a task to the receptionists to inform the patient and include the advice to seek medical attention if her symptoms don't improve or if she becomes worse. The advice to call the surgery in three days to check the results of the laboratory tests on the sample accompanies the already mentioned advice.

* * *

Ten to one and it is time to deal with the last four ring-backs still waiting on the screen.

Number twenty-nine is from twenty-two-year-old Cara, who has suffered from a headache for the last three days, in combination with cold symptoms. Cara thinks she has sinusitis and requests to be seen. I send a task to invite her for a sit-and-wait appointment at ten past four.

* * *

The thirtieth ring-back is from the mum of fifteen-year-old Melissa, who suffers from heavy and irregular periods. Mum would like her to be seen today. Again, I send a task to invite the patient for a sit-and-wait appointment, this one at twenty past four.

* * *

Then it is time for the last ring-back on the screen, thirteen-year-old Tilly has been self-harming and mum would like her to be seen today. There is no choice in this case and I send another task to over a sit-and-wait appointment for half-past four and ensure this will be a twenty-minute appointment. This problem cannot wait for a routine appointment. Within the task, I advise that if mum feels Tilly needs to be seen earlier than that, she should let us know.

* * *

Phew, finally I have finished.

It is then that I notice I did not respond to the fifth ring-back yet. The lady who had taken the morning off for an appointment. I feel horrible I missed Melanie's deadline even if her problem does not sound medically urgent to me. While I keep my fingers crossed Melanie won't complain about the delay, I send a task to the receptionists to invite her for a sit-and-wait appointment at ten to five.

With the morning ring-back list completed, I stretch, rub my neck and take a sip from my cold tea. With the visits waiting for me I will need to skip lunch. At least for now.

CHAPTER 9

Tuesday, 12:51 pm

Before I leave for my visits, I take more prescriptions and paperwork to reception and then go upstairs, use the bathroom and go to see the practice manager as she requested earlier. My stomach is grumbling, but it will need to wait for now.

Although I'm not sure what she needs to talk to me about, I suspect something is wrong as she often only asks to speak to us if a complaint has been received. After knocking on her door and entering, Angela greets me, "Busy day today?"

When I confirm it has been rather busy, Angela gets to the point, "Sorry, I'm not going to make your day any better. I received a complaint about you this morning. A patient you consulted today complains you were rude to him after already having left him waiting for over half an hour and then neglecting to give him the appropriate treatment for his problems."

Three guesses who that complaint is from. Why on earth do I still try? Whatever we do, it is never good enough. Sometimes it seems better to just say to a patient, you are right, I'm a bad doctor and I will put in my resignation right now. That is not actually true though. The majority of patients are very grateful for what we do, it is just patients like Darren, who make you doubt your conviction to your job. After reading his letter of complaint, I go over the consultation in my mind. Had I been rude? I'm sure I remained civil throughout the consultation, even when he called me all sort of names. If anyone was rude, I consider it to be Darren, but maybe I'm in the wrong here after all. How one person sees a situation is not always how another person sees it, right?

Should I have given in to Darren's pressure to prescribe antibiotics? Although it might have partially avoided the complaint, it would have been bad practice. Giving antibiotics when the situation does not require them, leads to bacteria developing a resistance to the antibiotics. These bacteria no longer respond to antibiotics and suddenly become killers. No, I'm not willing to enable this behaviour, complaint or no complaint.

Perhaps I should have been more compliant and not informed Darren we only allow one problem per consultation. However, patient education is important and if a patient is not aware of the fact he is supposed to book a longer appointment if he brings more than one problem to a consultation, he will continue to bring several complaints to one appointment in the future, 'to save time'. In fact, it leads exactly to what he also complained about, having had to wait for too long a period. Half an hour he had mentioned. I was certain it was less than half an hour. Unless, of course, Darren included the wait from the time he arrived at the surgery to his appointment time and the quarter of an hour he had to wait after his appointment time.

At the moment my mood has plummeted, I'm hungry and there is still a lot of work ahead of me today. Now, I will first need to get ready for the visits and deal with the work during the rest of the afternoon. And when I have a moment, I will need to respond to that complaint. Dutifully apologise for any upset I have caused him and for the rude behaviour I was not aware I displayed. Really, why do I still try?

* * *

I grab my bag and make sure all the necessary is present in the bag and move to reception.

"I'm off on my visits now, see you later."

Elaine looks up, "Thanks Dr Ellen, see you soon."

I exit via the back door and get into my car, then drive to the nursing home. After ringing the bell, it takes several minutes before someone answers the door and I stand shuffling my feet. Come on, I haven't got all day. Still, I realise they can't leave a resident in the middle of caring for him or her to answer the door.

"Afternoon, I'm here to visit," a quick check of my papers, "Joseph and Muriel."

The nurse leads me to the office and tells me that Joseph is on this side of the home, but Muriel lives on the other side.

"Tell me about Joseph."

"Well, Joseph is an eighty-nine-year-old man, who is more drowsy than usual. Over the last two days, he has been coughing, but he has not brought any phlegm up. I'm a little worried Joseph is too weak to bring anything up."

By now we reach his room and there is a strong and concentrated smell of urine in his room. "Have you checked his urine at all?"

"Well, no doctor, he does not pass a lot of urine at the moment."

Now, I'm getting a little more concerned, "Is he drinking?"

The nurse shakes her head, "Not much, I'm afraid, we need to encourage him to drink and even then he often refuses."

After I ask her to check his urine, I turn to the patient,

"Hello, Joseph, I'm Dr Ellen. Can I have a listen to your chest please?"

Joseph opens his eyes and smiles a little, "Okay doctor."

The nurse helps Joseph to sit up a little, so I can listen to his chest. "Thank you, that's fine. Your chest is clear."

She has tested his urine in the meantime and this shows signs of infection.

After leaving a prescription for antibiotics, advising Joseph to drink more fluids and asking the nurse to contact us if Joseph does not improve or if his condition worsens, she leads me to the connecting door of the nursing home. The nurse opens it and paces to the office on that side of the home.

Soon the nurse for that part of the home joins us and it is time to visit the next patient.

* * *

Muriel is a 101-year-old lady who is in the end-stages of dementia. She no longer has much understanding, does no longer recognise her family and speech is non-existent. She is bedbound and needs to be helped with all her care needs. Even eating and drinking is a struggle, at times she appears to have forgotten how to swallow and food will remain in her mouth for a long time.

When we enter the room, Muriel's eighty-nine-year-old daughter is visiting, "Afternoon doctor, thank you for seeing mum today."

Muriel has had a skin lesion on her forehead for a long time and this appears to be slowly getting bigger. The nursing home staff and daughter have deliberated for a long time but would like to find out what it is.

"Do you think it is skin cancer, doctor?"

After checking the lesion, it indeed appears to be one of the fairly innocent forms of skin cancer. It measures about half a centimetre in diameter and resembles what in medical terms is called a basal cell carcinoma. These type of tumours grow relatively slowly and don't spread, other than enlarging a little over time. It is unlikely this will cause Muriel any problems. The lesion is a bit unsightly, but it is unlikely to cause her any harm.

When I explain to the daughter and nurse what the lesion is, the daughter becomes slightly agitated, "I don't want mum to go to the hospital, doctor. Mum wouldn't be able to cope with that and it would upset her." The nurse nods and I agree with their assessment.

At this stage of Muriel's dementia, going to the hospital to be prodded and poked would be far more upsetting and harmful to her than leaving the lesion alone. We decide to observe and if there is any change in the situation or if the daughter decides she wishes a hospital opinion, after all, we can always review the situation.

The lesion will likely die with Muriel, but it won't kill her. Keeping her at the nursing home feels like the right option for her.

Then I leave to get back to the surgery again. By now it is already two in the afternoon and surgery is due to start at half-past two again.

* * *

At ten past two, I return to the surgery. I wave to the receptionist to let her know I'm back in the premises and make my way to the room. A box of prescriptions is waiting on my desk as well as a few prescriptions spread in a fan on my desk. This means these need to be signed first. These prescriptions have either been generated from the minor illness clinic by the nurse or urgent requests from patients. After logging back on, I notice another ten ring-backs arrived during my absence from the surgery and decide to first enter the details of the visits on the patients' notes. My stomach is still rumbling and I take my lunchbox out of my bag and take a bite every now and then while doing my work while also signing some of the prescriptions waiting.

When both visits are entered on the patients' notes, I turn my attention to the new ring-backs and put my sandwich to the side. Lunch will need to wait until I have taken care of my patients first. The thought of how silly that is crosses my mind for a moment. I always tell patients they can only look after others if they look after themselves first. A little hypocritical, isn't it?

CHAPTER 10

Tuesday, 2:20 pm

Now, I turn my attention to the thirty-eighth ring-back of the day. Mum has phoned about four-year-old Ellie, who has been sent home from nursery with a temperature. Ellie is also crying all the time. In response, I send a task to the receptionists to invite her for a sit-and-wait appointment at ten to five.

* * *

The thirty-ninth ring-back is from Alicia, a twenty-seven-year-old pregnant lady who suffers from morning sickness. She is currently about ten weeks pregnant and wants something for the morning sickness. Another task is on its way to the receptionists to offer a sit-and-wait appointment at five. This problem is not as simple as it seems, there are no medications licensed for treating morning sickness. We will need to explore her problems and discuss all options.

* * *

Next are three related ring-backs. Two-year-old twins Linda and Amy and their three-year-old brother Bobby. Mum has phoned because the twins have cold and cough symptoms and Bobby has a sore throat, she would like all three children to be seen today.

Three tasks are sent to the receptionists, one for each child for sit-and-wait appointments at ten past, quarter past and twenty past five. As they are all related and suffer from similar problems, I expect to be able to see to their problems relatively quickly. That is ring-back forty to forty-two sorted. On to the next one and I rub my neck as I click on the next patient's name.

* * *

The forty-third ring-back is from a new mum, concerned about her three-week-old Finlay, who suffers from colic. Mum would like him to be checked over. This task asks mum to attend for a half-past five sit-and-wait appointment with Finlay.

Next, I glance at the forty-fourth ring-back, twenty-year-old Adam, who suffers from cold symptoms, a cough, no temperature and no phlegm. I decide to leave this one for later, my first patient of the afternoon has arrived after all.

The forty-fifth ring-back is from Chrissy, a thirty-eight-year-old lady with heavy periods and I decide this can wait until later as well.

* * *

The forty-sixth ring-back is from eighteen-year-old Hayley, who wants to see the doctor about an unwanted pregnancy. This requires a face-to-face consultation and I send a task to invite her for a sit-and-wait appointment at twenty to six. Hopefully, I won't get a lot of other ring-backs requiring sit-and-wait appointments. The surgery doors close at six and the receptionists leave around that time too unless there is an emergency. We will have to wait to find out what the rest of the afternoon brings today.

* * *

Feeling the pressure of the waiting patients, I decide it is now time to start the afternoon surgery. Before I call the first patient in, I take the prescriptions to reception and find the file room lady Marilyn has some further paperwork waiting for me. On my way to the bathroom, I drop this off at my room, I will check it later. First, I will go to the bathroom to take care of my needs. To have the pressure of a full bladder while consulting patients is not conducive for paying attention to details.

In the hallway, I meet Deborah, "Can you come and have a look at another patient for me, please?"

After accompanying her back to her room, I see fifty-eight-year-old Malcolm. Malcolm has a leg ulcer, which is not healing very well. I turn to Deborah while I sense my eyebrows move up a little, "How long has it been like this?"

Deborah confirms the ulcer has been like this for a few weeks, "The ulcer responded well to the treatment given initially. However, over the last few days, maybe even a week, it has worsened again. What do you think? Would you like to give him some antibiotics or would you like to wait for the results of the swab?"

The ulcer does not appear to be infected at the moment, there is no surrounding redness. There also is no discharge from the ulcer, another sign infection is unlikely.

"Let's wait with antibiotics until we have the results of the swab. The ulcer has been worsening though, right?"

Deborah nods and Malcolm looks from Deborah to me and back again.

"Okay, I think it is time to refer Malcolm to the Tissue

Viability Service. Don't you agree?"

Deborah nods again and I then turn towards Malcolm, "As your ulcer is not healing as well as we would like to see, we feel we should refer you to the Tissue Viability Service. This service is the expert on poorly healing ulcers and they may be able to help the ulcer heal quicker. Are you happy for that to happen?"

Malcolm nods and Deborah agrees to arrange the referral.

After leaving Deborah's room, I nip into the toilet and then return to my room. It is time to get back to work again.

CHAPTER 11

Tuesday, 2:40 pm

My first patient of the afternoon is Laura, an eighty-five-year-old lady with known angina, who already has received three bypass operations in the past. Over the last year, she has seen the specialist several times for ongoing chest pains and they have concluded no further surgical intervention is possible. Instead, Laura's medications are adjusted when necessary to keep her symptoms under control as far as possible.

Today Laura has come to discuss her chest pains again.

"When it is cold or if I walk up the stairs, I still get these tight pains, doctor. Do you think it is time to increase my medication again?"

First, I glance at the screen to check her medication list. Yes, there is still room to increase her medication further. At least, there will be if she has no problems tolerating the medication.

"Have you had any problems with side-effects on the medication at all?"

Laura shakes her head, "No, these tablets seem to suit me just fine. They are nothing like those last ones the specialist tried me with." A smile appears on her face.

"Okay, let's increase the tablets a little further in that case." Again, I turn towards the computer, to give Laura a prescription for the increased dose of medication.

"Thank you so much, doctor." Laura stands up to leave the room, and as she does I ask Laura to return in a week for review.

I want to make sure the dose increase works for her and add the advice to ring for an ambulance if Laura has symptoms which do not respond to her GTN spray (medication to spray under the tongue to relieve the angina pain). Laura nods, opens the door and leaves.

* * *

I'm running behind slightly and the next patient comes in ten minutes after her appointment time. Meghan is a thirty-seven-year-old lady, who tells me about her depression today, "Life just isn't worth living any longer. I'm no good to anyone and everyone would be better off without me. Martin constantly tells me how worthless I am and he should know. Martin is the one who knows me best." Tears run down Meghan's face.

An iron fist grabs hold of my heart, "What do you mean, life isn't worth living? Have you ever considered doing anything to hurt yourself?" An uncomfortable feeling settles in my chest as though something has physically gotten hold of my heart and is squeezing it.

Meghan dissolves in a flood of tears and nods, "I keep a nice stock of tablets stored away for when I can no longer cope, for when the time is right. Martin does not realise. If he did, he would hit me so hard, I wouldn't even make it to the hospital."

Wait? What did she say? My heart seems to skip a beat, "Does Martin hit you?"

Still crying, Meghan nods again, "Yes, but it is my own fault. Martin only hits me if the food is not ready on time or if there are still creases in his shirt after I ironed it. Only if I haven't done things right or if I haven't done what I was supposed to do."

And she considers that to be normal? With difficulty, I push down the fury that seems to rise up in my body. It would not do to show this to Meghan. However much the thought of what she has to go through bothers me, it is not professional to show my anger over it. "But Meghan, that does not give him the right to hit you. That is not acceptable behaviour. You can choose to not accept that. There are services available for you to help you with this."

Meghan shakes her head, "No it is my fault Martin hits me. He told me so. I'm worthless and can't do anything right. Only by hitting me will I ever learn how to do things right."

I shake my head. Meghan sounds like she has been completely brainwashed. This should not be allowed to continue, but if Meghan won't accept my help, what is there left to do?

A sudden thought flashes through my mind. "Do you and Martin have any children?"

If there are children in the household something needs to happen. Social services will need to be involved if Meghan is not willing to take control of the situation and get out of her abusive relationship.

She shakes her head and continues to look at the hands clenched in her lap, "Martin says it's my fault. Three years ago I lost a baby. "Can't even carry a baby right", he says. Things got worse since."

Okay, I discovered most of the back story now. Even without her willingness to accept help – why is she here if not asking for help? – I need to look further into the suicidal thoughts she expressed.

"You mentioned the tablets earlier, Is there anything that stops you from taking those at the moment?"

"Yes, if I take them, Martin will be so mad with me. There won't be tea on the table when he gets home."

"And is there anything that would make you take them?"

Tears continue to run down Meghan's face as her hands fidget in her lap, "If I lost the baby again." I can only just hear the whispered words.

This makes the situation even worse than it was already. "Does Martin know you're pregnant?"

Meghan shakes her head and continues to stare down, her voice continues in a whisper, "If he found out, he would kick my stomach again until I lost the baby. I'm not worthy to be a mum, too worthless. But I don't want to lose the baby." Meghan's sobs worsen and I can't help but take hold of her hand in an attempt to comfort the distressed woman.

Something needs to be done. If Meghan returns home to her husband, there is a distinct risk she and the baby might not survive.

Again I try to persuade Meghan to accept help. Surely she must have wanted help for her to attend the surgery? There seems to be a deep desire to protect her unborn baby and I may be able to use that to convince her.

"This baby is important to you, isn't it?"

Meghan nods.

"How far would you be willing to go to protect it?"

She looks up, "Anything," then adds, "anything

within reason. I can't leave Martin. He will never allow it."

"Do you want to leave him?"

Another nod, "I've tried a few times. Last time was when I lost the baby three years ago. I was clumsy and tripped over Martin's foot at the top of the stairs, then fell down it. He blamed me for being careless and hit me when I lay at the bottom of the stairs, then kicked my stomach. My clumsiness killed the baby, but I blamed Martin for a while and I ran away and stayed with my mum for a few weeks. When he told mum what I had done, she told me I should own up to my mistakes and go back to my husband. That I was unreasonable and Martin deserved better from me. I went home again that same day, I had no other choice."

Whoa! Her mum kicked her out after she had left Martin previously instead of standing up for her daughter? How manipulative was this guy? Or how blind was Meghan's mother?

"So, what would you like to do now?" Judging by Meghan's words, she was on the threshold of making a major decision regarding her future. A decision that could save the life of Meghan and her unborn baby. Still, Meghan's words regarding the pills remained in the back of my mind. Referral to the crisis team for assessment of her suicidal ideation might be necessary as well as referral to the domestic abuse centre.

"I don't know. Sometimes I want to leave Martin and never come back. But where can I go? Mum would just send me back home. Dad died years ago and my sister lives too far away. She has her own family to care for and does not need me to make her life worse. Anyway, Martin would find me. He will always find me."

As I move to the filing cabinet and take out the details for the domestic abuse centre, a little hope of a better life for Meghan and her unborn child flickers inside me. I hand the details to Meghan and she meets my eyes, "Do you really think these people can help me, doctor?"

"Yes, I think they can. The centre has helped a lot of women in a similar position and they can help you as well if you wish. No one is worthless, we all serve some role in this world. Don't let anyone tell you you're worthless, because they are wrong."

Will this be enough? Should I refer her to the crisis team as well?

"Now, if the centre helps you, how do you feel about those tablets you've stored away?"

A sheepish smile takes hold of Meghan's face, "I don't think they will be needed in that case, doctor. They would hurt the baby, wouldn't they?"

I nod, "Yes, they would certainly hurt the baby."

"Then I'll get rid of them as soon as I get home."

"So, what are your plans?"

"Martin won't be home until eight tonight. After I get home, I'll get rid of the tablets, pack a bag and see these people. I'm going to leave Martin, this time for good." A hopeful sparkle is in her eyes as a watery smile settles on her face.

Hope blooms in my heart and I hope Martin doesn't get home unexpectedly, "If you ever need to talk, you know where to find me. Also, if there ever is a time where you feel like you want to hurt yourself, please, don't suffer on your own, speak to someone instead."

Meghan promises she will, hugs me and leaves with a hopeful expression on her face. Please let her be okay. Maybe I will have made a bit of a difference today. It is all I can hope for.

* * *

The consultation with Meghan understandably took far longer than the allotted ten minutes. Thirty-five minutes after Meghan entered my room, she left. By now I'm running forty-five minutes behind and I feel horrible and guilty about this, but hopeful of a better life for Meghan. The delay was, however, unavoidable. Meghan required the extra time and I'm glad I allowed her that time. After this consultation, I also need a little time for housekeeping. Looking after my own feelings is important too. If I am upset and don't calm down before I see the next patient, this could lead to making mistakes.

So, I sit back in the chair, close my eyes and take a few deep breaths. Then I buzz for the next patient.

* * *

Thirty-four-year-old Shelly sashays in and I apologise for running late due to an emergency I had to deal with.

"Don't worry, it's fine. These things happen."

What a breath of fresh air! Too often patients don't accept emergencies can pop up and react aggressively instead.

Shelly tells me about the painful elbow she has suffered from for the last ten weeks, which has gradually worsened.

On examination, I confirm a right tennis elbow, which is an irritation of the insertion of the tendons at the elbow, and Shelly's expression turns confused, "But I don't play tennis, doctor."

After explaining this is just a name and not necessarily relates to playing tennis, advising her to take pain relief if needed and informing Shelly this problem may take a few months to settle, she leaves and promises to return if her symptoms worsen or don't improve.

* * *

The next patient is twenty-six-year-old Julie, who has come with her partner. They have tried for the last year to conceive and are now getting concerned that something may be wrong. Generally, the rule is to start investigations after trying for eighteen months with no success.

As they appear genuinely concerned and distressed, I agree to arrange blood tests for Julie and a sperm count for her partner, who is also registered at our practice. Once the results are back, we can decide what the next step should be.

It is not very frequent GPs get the chance to see a patient before they get pregnant and I take this opportunity to give her some preconception advice, or advice before getting pregnant if you wish. After advising smoking cessation, drinking little to no alcohol, weight loss, Julie is in the obese range, and taking folic acid from now on, I move on to check if she is on any medication which might be unsafe for the baby.

The repeat prescription screen shows an interesting

item which was last issued a month ago. It is the contraceptive pill.

"Can I just check, Julie, are you still taking the pill?"

Wide-open eyes look at me, "Yes, of course. Shouldn't I?"

Aha, the problem seems to have been found, "Well, it is a great idea to take the pill. But only if you don't want to get pregnant. If you want to get pregnant, you should stop taking it."

Her partner turns towards her, "See. I told you so. But no, you insisted you needed to take the pill to regulate your periods." He crosses his arms and faces slightly away from Julie.

After advising to stop taking the pill, leaving the blood tests and sperm count for now and agreeing they will return if they still have problems conceiving after trying for another year to eighteen months, they leave. I'm left wondering how people can forget about the simple things at times.

* * *

Now it's time to move on to the next patient, twenty-two-year-old Tim, who has suffered from a sore throat for three days. On examination his throat looks fine, no redness, no swollen tonsils and his glands are fine. Tim's temperature is normal at 37.2. After general advice and telling him to return if his symptoms worsen, it is time to turn my attention to the next patient. At least this gives me a chance to reduce the amount of time I'm running behind.

* * *

Fortunately, my next patient is an easy one as well. Twenty-year-old Millie requests to have a repeat of her contraceptive pill. Millie was started on this six months ago and is not due the annual pill check yet. I issue the prescription and advise her that she can request the prescription without seeing a GP first, with the exception of the annual pill check, which will be due in six months.

* * *

Happy I have reduced the amount of time I'm running behind by another five minutes and to now be only twenty-five minutes behind, I call in the next patient.
Thirty-five-year-old Vicky is a mother of three active children who has come for review of her depression. She is still feeling down, although things are improving slightly. There is a questionnaire we use to check the severity and the progress of a patient's depression, the PHQ-9. which is a list of nine

questions. Each answer is scored and can get zero to three points. A score of twenty-seven would be the worst score possible, the patient being suicidal and high-risk to act on his or her feelings. Vicky's score has reduced from twelve to seven since the last time she was seen four weeks ago.

We agree to give her a sick note for another two weeks and discuss the possibility of returning to work on a phased return after that.

"Do you really think I may be ready to go back to work then?" Vicky looks a little concerned.

"If you continue to improve as you have done over the last few months, yes, I think you might be. But let's wait until next time before making any decisions on that, shall we?"

Vicky looks a little more relaxed now and leaves the room with a smile on her face.

* * *

The next patient is eighty-five-year-old Phyllis, who has come for a pessary fit. Phyllis saw me a week ago with symptoms of urinary incontinence and we discussed options to treat the prolapse found at that time. Phyllis preferred to try the ring pessary in the first instance and after having given her a prescription for one, she returns today with the pessary.

Again I go over the procedure with her and she disappears behind the curtain to remove her underpants and climb on the bed. Phyllis is able to relax quite well, and the pessary is fitted easily and with no problems. Although we usually allow twenty minutes for a pessary change, this is completed within ten minutes today and we agree she will only need a ten-minute appointment for this procedure next time.

Fortunately, this has allowed me to catch up a little further. Not that I will be able to catch up fully. Phyllis' appointment was due at twenty to four and it was already two past four when she came in.

* * *

By now it's twelve past four and before seeing the first extra patients of the afternoon, I glance at a few of the new ring-backs received.

The first one on the list to process, the forty-seventh of today, is from eighty-three-year-old Margaret, who suffers from a painful knee due to known osteoarthritis. She wants to get some advice on her pain relief.

Now, I pick up the phone and call Margaret. After a short chat, she tells me she takes co-codamol, a combination of codeine and paracetamol, for her pain. She has no side-effects and takes one tablet a day as she is worried she might overdose on them. After reassuring her she can take up to two tablets at a time up to four times a day if the pain is severe, she hangs up promising to take the painkillers a bit more often if she needs them. Margaret will contact us again if she has any problems after doing so or if the tablets give her problems.

* * *

The next ring-back is from fifty-two-year-old Robert, a known alcoholic who tends to phone us a few times a week. Generally, he is intoxicated when he rings and slurring his words. His request sounds simple enough, he wants help. He claims to be housebound, but is still observed frequenting the shop to buy his alcohol, and today Robert wants to be admitted for his depression. "Life is not worth living" is his usual phrase. However, if any help is offered, he refuses it.

Already aware this call will take a long time again, the last time I spoke to him I was on the line for over an hour, I decide to leave it till the end of surgery.

* * *

The last ring-back I check before seeing the extra

patients booked in for this afternoon, is from thirty-seven-year-old Jonathan. He uses paracetamol for a painful back and has forgotten to put his repeat prescription request in on time. Now he has been shouting at the receptionists, demanding a repeat prescription for this. This should have been ready two minutes before he asked for it, obviously. And without a doubt, it is the fault of the receptionists and the doctor it has not been done yet. I do not happen to agree with Jonathan's view on things. And I certainly don't agree with how he is treating the members of my team.

Paracetamol is a medication which is also available over the counter, in other words, Jonathan can buy them at the pharmacy or even at the supermarket without a prescription. His request for an urgent prescription is therefore unreasonable and I send a task to the receptionists to advise Jonathan to buy them himself while awaiting the prescription to be processed in the usual manner. Hopefully, he won't cause my receptionists too much grief over this.

Otherwise, we can expect yet another complaint to come our way. However, I'm not going to give in to emotional blackmail and if he is abusive towards the girls, he can expect a warning letter himself. I'm sure the girls will let me know if he is abusive towards them.

CHAPTER 12

Tuesday, 4:21 pm

And then it's time to see the first extra patient of the afternoon. Before I move on to the next patient, however, I pay a quick visit to the bathroom.

The first extra patient is twenty-two-year-old Cara, who was one of the last ring-backs this morning. Cara has suffered from a headache for the last three days and also suffers from cold symptoms.

"This headache has not wanted to leave me for the last three days, doctor. And it is worse when I change position. Then it feels like a brick tries to fall through my forehead, especially when I lean forward. And my snot is a horrible green colour."

While I take the digital thermometer out of the drawer, I turn towards Cara again, "Okay, let's examine you."

She has a slight temperature of 37.8, green nasal discharge and when I tap her forehead, she nearly hits the roof.

"You appear to have sinusitis. Are you allergic to any antibiotics?"

Fortunately, she has no allergies, but Cara is on the combined contraceptive pill, I notice.

"Do you still use the pill?"

Cara nods and pulls a face as the movement has worsened her headache again.

"Antibiotics interfere with the effectiveness of the pill. You should, therefore, take extra precautions for the week you are on the pill and the week after if you don't wish to have any unexpected surprises."

After taking the prescription from the printer and signing it, I turn to Cara again, "Try steam inhalation too, this may help with the pain and to speed the recovery on a little. If your symptoms don't improve after a few days or if they worsen, you should seek medical attention again."

Cara thanks me and leaves. Now it is time to move on to the next task.

* * *

The next patient is fifteen-year-old Melissa who attends with her mum because of her irregular and heavy periods. Although it is easy to just take what a patient tells us for granted, I delve into the problem a little deeper. Everyone is different and often a person's interpretation of what is and what is not normal deviates from what we consider being normal.

"So Melissa, your mum tells me your periods are irregular and heavy. Is that true?"

Melissa looks down at her hands and nods. It does not appear she is happy to be here.

"Tell me, what are they like, how long is there usually between the start of one period and the start of the next one."

Melissa glances up for a moment, "I dunno. Like every five weeks or something, I guess."

Mum interrupts, a determined look in her eyes, "See, I told you, Melissa is irregular. She does not have a period every four weeks as you would expect, she has one every five weeks instead. That's not normal now, is it?"

As I glance over to mum, I wonder how best to let her know every five weeks is regular and normal without upsetting mum in the process. Carefully, I explain every woman is different and even if someone has a period every three, four or five weeks, this is still considered normal. Hardly any woman works like clockwork and if a period comes regularly, give or take a few days either side, this is still normal.

"But, her periods are really heavy. Surely you can do something about that, doctor?"

Again I turn towards Melissa, "How heavy are your periods, Melissa? Do you need to change your pad often?"

"I dunno, once in the morning, once in the afternoon and before I go to bed, I guess." Melissa is still looking down and avoiding eye contact.

That is not what we consider very heavy, "Do you lose any clots while you're on your period?"

Both mum's and Melissa's eyes shoot wide-open as they stare at me like I've asked them if she is birthing an alien every time. Mum takes a deep breath, "But surely that is not normal, is it? I mean, I spot for two or three days and always have done. Changing as much as Melissa does can't be right, can it?"

Again I explain most women need to change that often and a lot of women even more frequently than Melissa does. It takes some work, but finally, the message appears to filter through and now reassured, Melissa and her mother leave and I turn my attention to the next patient on my list.

* * *

Now it's time to see thirteen-year-old Tilly, who has been self-harming and whose mum is concerned about her. I would be if Tilly was my daughter.

Mum enters the room and immediately starts a tirade,

"I need Tilly to be seen today by a psychiatrist. She needs to be admitted. What if she kills herself?"

As I turn toward Tilly and her mother, I indicate the chairs, "Why don't you take a seat and we can talk about what is happening?"

Both take a seat and Tilly keeps her hands in her lap, staring at them and fidgeting. Mum's face looks like thunder, "My daughter is self-harming and you want to," she makes air quotes with her fingers, "talk about it? Talking about it won't help. Something needs to be done to stop Tilly from hurting herself. You need to get Tilly the help she needs." Tears run down mum's face and Tilly continues with her fidgeting and has yet to make eye contact with me. Are those tears of despair or anger? Mum looks like she wants to attack me and I try to take a deep breath without her noticing.

"Can you tell me what has been happening?"

"Tilly's PE teacher phoned me four days ago. Mrs Blake explained how she had seen cuts on Tilly's upper legs during PE that day and was concerned about it." Mum's eyes shoot angry fire at me and spittle shoots from her mouth, "I tried to get an appointment for Tilly ever since. This should have been dealt with as an emergency but instead we were made to wait! How can you call yourselves a caring practice if you don't offer an appointment when people need one? This is totally unacceptable and I'm considering taking this to our MP." After leaving her to rant for a while, Mum calms down a little, "Well, don't you think it is unacceptable to be kept waiting this long?"

How can I defuse this situation and get Tilly the attention and help she needs?

"I am sorry to have kept you waiting such a long time but the important thing is Tilly is here today and we need to find out what is happening to help her with this." As I turn towards Tilly to engage her in the conversation, mum appears to be angry I dared move away from her. Still, I want to get Tilly's thoughts on the matter. Without knowing what Tilly thinks about it and why she feels she self-harms, we won't get very far.

"Is that right, Tilly? Have you been cutting yourself?" A slight nod follows, but she has yet to speak a word. "Can you tell me how long you have been cutting yourself for?"

Tilly shrugs but still does not speak.

"A few days?" Another shrug, "a few weeks?" yet another shrug, "a few months?" Tilly gives a tiny nod. Okay, we are slowly getting somewhere. Although Tilly is reluctant to speak and take part in the conversation, we now have confirmation she has been cutting herself for a few months.

After persisting a while longer, Tilly finally speaks and tells us she started cutting herself about five months ago. Her friends told her she was ugly and did not deserve to be in the same class as them. Now, Tilly usually sits on her own and even then they find her and kick her bag, pull her hair followed by an "oops, sorry, didn't realise you were there, invisible girl" and they even pushed her onto the street as a joke. This would be followed by giggling from the group of girls around and shouts of "Whoa, Tilly, you may be ugly, but that is no reason to throw yourself under the bus."

Mum's eyes open wider and wider during the conversation, mouth open in surprise. The anger appears to have dissolved a little and concern and amazement fill her face instead.

Tilly's so-called friends have also told her she should just kill herself as nobody likes her, anyway. She should stop wasting the air they breathe. Once Tilly gets started, there is no stopping her and tears run down her face.

"But why didn't you tell me?" It is difficult to be certain if mum is simply shocked or if she is furious with Tilly for not telling her about the bullying at school.

"Have you spoken to anyone about this Tilly, to a teacher perhaps?"

Tilly shakes her head, "I can't. That will only make it worse. And they only do it when there is no one around to see it."

Bit by bit the story emerges and like so many other people who self-harm, this is an outward manifestation of the pain they feel inside. After a lot of persuasion, Tilly allows me to examine the cuts, which are indeed limited to her upper legs, shallow and fortunately unlikely to leave much scarring.

We discuss alternative ways to cope with the problem and mum will speak to the teachers and counsellor at school and if no help is forthcoming, consider transferring Tilly to a different school.

Tilly promises to talk to mum more and to stop cutting if possible. If this is found to be too difficult, they will return for a referral to counselling to help Tilly cope with her problems.

When they leave, I'm left fuming. I hate bullies, they do so much damage to the fragile people around them.

After a deep breath, I continue with the heavy workload.

* * *

The next emergency patient is the lady with hair loss I almost forgot about. Fortunately, she was able to accept the afternoon appointment and I hope she is not too angry with me for not being more accommodating towards her.

When Melanie enters, she appears extremely annoyed. I'm running a little late and she is seen six minutes after the scheduled appointment time.

"This surgery is rubbish. There are never any appointments available if I need one."

Although I am tempted to point out several appointments were available last week when Melanie claimed there weren't, I hold my tongue.

"When I phoned this morning, the receptionist told me you would ring-back within an hour."

I am quite certain the receptionists would never make a promise like that unless there was an emergency and in that case they would warn me about this.

"Instead, I was kept waiting for hours and when I then finally get an appointment for this afternoon, you keep me waiting another half an hour."

Again I am tempted to point out I'm only six minutes late, but I bite my tongue again.

Melanie takes a deep breath before continuing, "This practice never does anything to help patients. I could have been dead already." Dead of hair loss? Really? That is not something I ever encountered before. "To be honest, I should put a complaint in and I think I will. You seriously neglect my needs." Melanie pauses for a moment, "Actually, perhaps I should just go to the paper with this. That will teach you to treat people the way they should be treated. You are a disgrace."

Spittle shoots from Melanie's mouth and lands on my cheek and I need to restrain myself from wiping it away. Such an action would no doubt infuriate her further and I already upset her enough as it is. Instead, I take a deep breath, hoping to control myself before addressing Melanie, "I am very sorry to keep you waiting and to hear you were unable to get a suitable appointment. To be honest, I was not aware I was running behind half an hour already, but I do apologise for the inconvenience I've caused you. But now you are here, perhaps you can tell me what seems to be the problem." Oops, I almost pointed out I was only six minutes late and that really might have blown up the situation.

"Well, it is like this doctor. Over the last two months I've been losing loads of hair. I'm convinced I'm going bald and you need to do something about that."

"When you say you're losing hair, how much is this? Are there clumps on the pillow, any bald patches you have noticed?" While I glance at Melanie, she appears to own a full head of hair, but I have not yet properly examined her.

"No, not clumps on the pillow, but there is a handful

DIARY OF A FEMALE GP

of hair in the hairbrush when I brush it after washing my hair. Surely that is not normal. I'm convinced my hair feels thinner as well."

After examining her hair, there is no sign of any bald patches or even thinning of her hair.

"How about organising a few blood tests to rule out some common and treatable causes of hair loss?"

Melanie looks at me expectantly and I forge forward, "The hair loss does not appear to be too bad at the moment. I can't see any bald patches and suspect everything is going to turn out just fine."

However, my reassurances fall on deaf ears as Melanie again appears thunderous. When she leaves after my advice to return if things don't improve or if they get worse, I wonder if I will have another complaint on my desk in the next few days. Judging by Melanie's thunderous face, it appears likely.

* * *

Before seeing my next patient, I fill my cup with tea again. The need to do some 'housekeeping' is obvious. I need to calm myself down enough to be able to cope with the next patient in an appropriate manner and at the moment I am anything but calm. After taking a deep breath, I stand up and go through the first part of the kata I learned at last week's karate lesson. The concentration this takes helps me to calm down further and now I can call in the next patient.

Twenty-seven-year-old Alicia is ten weeks pregnant and suffers from severe morning sickness. Although she is sick several times a day, she generally is able to keep food and fluids down and this is a positive sign.

"But won't it harm the baby if I don't keep food down?" Anxious eyes glance back towards me as Alicia waits for an answer.

After I reassure Alicia that babies will withdraw all the nutrients from mum, even if she has none to spare, and the baby is quite safe under the circumstances, Alicia still requests medication to stop the sickness. "It is horrible doctor, I hate being sick. Can't you give me something to stop this?"

Instead I explain the problem with medication in pregnancy, "As long as you are able to keep some food and at least fluids down, it would be better not to give you anything for it. Unfortunately none of the anti-sickness medication is recommended for pregnancy. The majority of this medication carries the advice to avoid in pregnancy and the ones that don't still advise to use only if unavoidable. I would advise you to continue without medication if possible."

Reluctantly Alicia nods, "If it's not safe for the baby, I will persist. It is horrible though."

Next I tell her about a few things she can do to help her morning sickness, "Often the morning sickness is not too bad if you ensure your stomach is never fully empty. Having frequent small meals, ginger biscuits and drinking flat cola may also help. Most women also find the morning sickness disappears after thirteen weeks of pregnancy so that is something to look forward to."

Alicia agrees that it is better to continue as she is now. After all, she is already ten weeks pregnant. She does not want to take anything that might harm the baby and I agree with that statement.

* * *

Now Lindsay saunters in, a buggy with her two-year-old twins in front of her while her three-year-old son holds on to the buggy. Linda and Amy and their three-year-old brother Bobby are coughing and spluttering as they enter the room.

Linda is smiling and appears happy. The cough and cold have been present for a few days now and she has continued to eat well. When I examine Linda, her temperature is 37.8, a mild temperature only. Her ears, throat and chest are normal and she has a few small glands in her neck. Linda's breathing and heart rate are normal too and there is nothing to make me excessively concerned.

After reassuring mum and advising her about seeking medical attention if she worsens, it is time to look at the next twin.

* * *

Next it is Amy's turn. She is active and smiling and wants to run around the consultation room. Amy has already climbed out of the buggy and is now opening cupboards and drawers as she struts around the room, mum running after her.

"Don't Amy. Naughty. Nooo!" Mum has her hands full with her two-year-old. Bobby still stands next to the buggy, stopping Linda from climbing out too.

"So, how long has Amy been poorly for?" Not that Amy appears to be poorly.

"Just like Linda she started about three days ago. Coughing day and night, a temperature and very snotty. Could you just check her over, please?"

Now, I proceed to examine Amy. Mum holds her still on her lap. The examination is similar to the one for her sister. Her throat is fine, she has a temperature of 37.6 and her chest is clear. Her right ear looks fine, but the left drum is red. Amy's breathing and heart rate are fine too, a small wonder after the running she has done around my room.

"Amy has a middle ear infection on the left. Is she allergic to any antibiotics?"

Mum reassures me none of the children have any known allergies and I hand her a prescription for antibiotics to treat the problem, "Please book another appointment if Amy does not improve over the next few days or if she gets any worse."

* * *

Now it is 3-year-old Bobby's turn. His history is similar to his sisters'.

"Bobby started with a cold about five days ago. So far, his cough is not getting any better and nursery asked me to pick him up today as they felt he was unwell."

Bobby is clingy and does not want to let go of his mum, while the twins need to be kept from exploring drawers and cupboards and lifting textbooks from the bookcase. Textbooks which are far too heavy for them. Amy has managed to escape from the buggy too.

Bobby's temperature is 38.3, and he looks more ill than his sisters. His throat and ears are okay and his breathing seems a little fast.

"Can I have a listen to your chest, Bobby?"

He looks at me and gives a small nod. When I place the stethoscope on his chest, I can hear a few crackles on the right side and his heart rate and breathing are slightly faster than would be expected in a well child. Not that fast an admission would be necessary, though.

"Bobby needs some antibiotics too, he has a chest infection," I tell Lindsay and she nods.

"I thought he was worse than the twins, he just isn't like his usual self."

Bobby also has no allergies and after giving him a prescription for antibiotics and advising mum to return if Bobby worsens or does not improve, the family leaves.

* * *

By now it is half-past five, and I have caught up on the time I ran behind. The next patient is three-week-old Finlay, who comes with his mum.

"I can't do this anymore doctor, I'm at my wit's end."

Finlay is her first baby and continuously seems to cry from ten at night till about two in the morning. During the day he cries a lot too, but that is easier to cope with. However, as this has kept her awake at night, Ellie is now exhausted and coping during the day is more difficult too.

"When Finlay starts to cry at night, I just can't settle him. Whatever I do, he only keeps screaming. Something must be wrong. Please check him and find out what is wrong." Tears roll down her face and there are large dark circles underneath mum's eyes, evidence of her poor sleep. When examination only shows a healthy baby boy and I reassure mum, she calms down a little, "I was so worried."

I explain that Finlay most likely suffers from the three-month colic, something that usually resolves after three months. When I ask about support, mum confirms that her parents and her partner are supportive and she will speak to them to make sure she can also get some rest.

Armed with a prescription for Infacol to help with the colic and the promise she can come back if things don't improve or if they get worse, mum leaves with Finlay, looking much happier than when she came in.

* * *

Now it's time to see Hayley, an eighteen-year-old, who wants to see me about an unwanted pregnancy. Unfortunately, I am the only doctor in the surgery who is willing to refer patients for a termination. Although I would never consider one for myself, it is my belief a woman has the right to make a decision about that herself. That is, after ensuring the woman is aware of all the options open to her and informing her she can change her mind at any stage. Unlike many people believe, a termination is not an easy decision or the easy route. I have seen too many women regretting a termination in later years to ever consider it that.

Hayley ambles in, her head dipped down. After offering her a seat and asking what I can do for her, Hayley starts her story.

"I don't know what to do, doctor. My period was late, and I did a test a few days ago, hoping against hope it would be negative. But, of course, it was positive and now I don't know what to do. There is no way I can cope with a baby at the moment. I'm about to start university in September and, well it's just not the right time in my life." Hayley starts to cry, "I never expected I would ask you this, but can you arrange a termination for me, please?"

From what Hayley has said so far, it is obvious she does not really want to make this decision.

"When did you find out about the pregnancy and do you have any idea how far along you are?"

Hayley glances up, "My period should have come a week ago, the test was done two days ago."

"Have you really thought about this decision? This is not an easy decision to make and you need to be certain this is the right thing for you. No one can tell you if this is the right decision, only you can."

Again she starts to cry, "Well, I didn't tell you earlier,

but this was not only unplanned," Hayley sobs even more, "But..., but..., I was raped a month ago. I don't consider I can cope with being reminded about that my entire life."

Oh, Hayley, what a horrible thing to happen to you. I pull myself together, "As long as you feel this is the right thing for you to do, that is fine. There is no need to hurry a decision, there is still time to ponder it over for a while longer if you wish. But, ultimately, the decision is yours and yours alone. Don't ever think we will judge you for your decision. And, if you find that it was more difficult than you anticipated and you find it difficult to cope with your decision, remember, we're still here and happy to help and support you."

There is, however, something else that needs to be addressed. "Did you report the rape?"

Hayley shakes her head and bites her lip, "No, it was one of my friends and I don't want to make matters worse. Jim will only say I was happy enough to have sex with him and there is no way to prove I wasn't. We were alone at the time and although I did tell Jim to stop, it will be my word against his."

After discussing this a little longer, Hayley sticks with the decision not to report the rape. She is also, understandably, still convinced it is best to have a termination. I give Hayley a little credit card sized card with the number for BPAS (British Pregnancy Advisory Service) and ask her to book her appointment, stressing she can change her mind at any time she wishes. Next, I also advise Hayley to see the sexual health clinic to rule out any sexually transmitted diseases if she decides not to report the rape. Hayley has quite enough to work through as it is. After offering support and a willing ear if she needs it, Hayley leaves and I take a deep breath to collect myself again. Another emotionally charged appointment. Sometimes it appears the day is filled with them.

* * *

Hayley was the last emergency patient booked in. Now only ring-backs remain on the screen and I ring the patients back, one after the other.

The forty-fourth ring-back is one I put to the side to sort out after surgery, twenty-year-old Adam. When I ask him to tell me what the problem is, he starts talking.

"Well, I have had this cold and cough for a few days and I wondered if I had a chest infection and needed antibiotics."

After asking him about further symptoms, Adam continues, "No, I'm not breathless and I'm not bringing anything up. It's just this horrible phlegm at the back of my throat that sticks there and doesn't want to move anywhere. At night this seems to be worse and keeps me awake, just keeps tickling in the back of my throat." Adam denies a temperature or feeling unwell.

When I check the clock, it is already a quarter to six and there is no way Adam could get to the surgery before it closes at six. Besides, Adam is still at work, which is over half an hour away from the surgery.

"Okay Adam, it sounds like you have a cold. Try some steam inhalation and if your symptoms don't improve or if they get worse, you should book an appointment and see someone about them."

Adam is happy with this solution and it is time to move on to the next ring-back.

* * *

Next on the list is thirty-eight-year-old Chrissy, "It's my heavy periods, doctor. Over the last six months, they are heavier than usual, some have clots in them and they also last a little longer than they used to. In the past, they only lasted about three days, but now they last five days."

Chrissy is not on the pill as she was sterilised and she is currently not in a relationship. She is adamant there is no risk of pregnancy as she has not had intercourse in the last three years. We discuss the options. Ideally, we would book her in for an appointment in routine, arrange a few blood tests or we might try some medication to hopefully reduce the heavy periods by reducing the clots.

Chrissy is not keen to take time off to visit a doctor at the moment and would like to try medication. After issuing a prescription and informing Chrissy she can pick this up in the morning, I advise her to see a doctor for review if the symptoms do not improve or if they worsen and turn my attention to the next ring-back.

* * *

The fiftieth item on the list is a urine sample for a thirty-seven-year-old lady. Millie is not pregnant, has no allergies, does not suffer from urine infections generally and is not on any other medication. The sample is suggestive of infection and I issue a prescription for antibiotics and send a task to the receptionists to ask them to inform the patient of this.

Would this have happened nowadays, I would not issue any prescription yet. The guidance has recently changed, and the advice is to await the results of the laboratory examination prior to prescribing unless the patient is symptomatic. Millie's urine sample would, therefore, not qualify for a prescription for antibiotics.

* * *

The next ring-back is for an eighty-seven-year-old resident of a nursing home. Marjorie has tripped and fallen and complains of a painful hip; she is unable to bear weight on it. The carer has asked if I can come and check Marjorie over. Instead, I send a task to the receptionists, and an instant message to alert them to the task, to advise the home to take the lady to casualty to rule out a fractured hip. There is nothing I can do about that if I visit and the outcome would likely be the same.

* * *

The fifty-second ring-back of today is a visit request from thirty-three-year-old Michelle, who has a roast in the oven and wants me to visit to check her thumb. When she put the roast in the oven, she burnt it and put the thumb under the tap straight afterwards. Although she is adamant the burn is not bad, she insists I need to visit her. Michelle is not housebound, but as she has a roast in the oven, she can't come to the surgery, hence her request.

After explaining that a roast in the oven is not an appropriate reason to receive a visit and that if she wishes to be seen, she should have made an appointment instead or, if she is concerned about the burn, she should attend A&E for an assessment of it.

Michelle is still not happy but reluctantly accepts.

"Well, if you're too lazy to come out and visit, which I might add is your duty to do if requested, I have no choice but to go to A&E."

Hopefully, that is not yet another complaint, but come on, demanding a visit because your roast is in the oven? Really?

Anyway, a GP does not have a duty to visit a patient unless the doctor considers the patient needs to be seen face-to-face to assess the problem, and the patient is housebound. In this case that does not apply. Michelle is not housebound and if the burn needs assessing, it would be more appropriate for her to attend the casualty department.

A text comes in from Martin, "Are you still working?" After returning his text with "Sorry, still another hour at least," I get back to work. If I don't make a move on with work, it will only last longer before I can return home. But I wish I could leave already.

* * *

Finally, the end appears to be in sight. Only two more ring-backs left. No more ring-backs are likely to pop up as it is already two minutes past six and the lines have been switched over to out of hours by now.

The next ring-back is from fifty-six-year-old Jack, who has suffered from an itchy rash for the last two years. Jack has told the receptionist his creams are not helping, and he considers this to be an urgent reason to be seen today. His call was received five minutes ago. It appears Jack only decided this was urgent five minutes ago.

When I phone him and ask why he considers this problem to be an emergency today, he tells me it is urgent because he has run out of his creams and he needs another prescription. He only uses E45, a moisturiser, for his eczema. This cream is also available over the counter at a pharmacy or even a supermarket and when I inform him of this, he is not a happy bunny. "But you should do me a prescription for that now."

I promise to do the prescription, which he can pick up tomorrow and suggest if his symptoms are bad enough, he buys the cream at the supermarket to help him while he waits to get his prescription.

As the call ends, I sense I have yet another unhappy customer. Am I really that unreasonable? Or are there too many patients with unreasonable expectations?

* * *

And then it is time to move on to the last ring-back of the day. The ring-back I pushed to the end, dreading to need to speak to him. Before I pick up the phone to speak to Robert, I first go to the bathoom. Robert will likely keep me on the line for at least half an hour and my bladder is already bursting.

At ten past six, I pick up the phone and call Robert. When he answers the phone, he is slurring the words, and it is obvious Robert is drunk once again. Generally, Robert only phones when drunk. During the infrequent periods he controls his drinking or is sober for a few weeks on end, he does not contact us at all. I take a deep breath and brace myself for the call ahead.

"You need to help me, I can't go on like this. I need to stop drinking, but I've had a setback and now I'm drinking again. It's too expensive, can't afford this. Aren't there any benefits I can get?"

Robert keeps talking and asking questions. A headache is trying to take hold as I try to concentrate on what he says and to make out the heavily slurred words. This is not an easy task.

"Really, there should be benefits for people like me. I can't afford to drink, but with benefits I could. Then I wouldn't need to bother you."

Robert continues to talk and I only make out some of what he spurts out. Next, he moves on to needing help to stop drinking.

"When I tried the alcohol services, they told me you have to ask them to do a home visit. You know I never leave the house, I just can't."

The fact the receptionists have seen Robert rush to the shop to get more alcohol passes through my mind, but I decide not to contradict him.

"So, how do you get the alcohol, Robert?"

He tells me a friend gets this for him sometimes and he can just manage to get to the corner shop to get some more alcohol.

Now Robert starts to cry, "What is there for me in life, anyway? My wife and kids left me, I have no one. Mum no longer wants to know me, nor do my brother and sisters. My kids never visit. And that's not right. That shouldn't be right. No one cares, maybe I should simply drink myself to death. That would teach everyone."

It is difficult to find a place to interrupt him, he simply does not stop talking. When I offer to refer him to the alcohol services or get the community mental health team to contact him, he refuses as usual. He reassures me he won't kill himself, "I'm too much of a coward for that, anyway."

Finally three-quarters of an hour later, we end the call after Robert hangs up on me. When I phone back, a friend answers the phone. She informs me she has arrived two minutes ago and that Robert is now asleep. She'll make sure he is okay and if needed she will contact someone for him overnight.

* * *

Finally! It is five to seven and I hear the cleaners hoovering the hallway and rooms around me. There is a knock on the door and they ask if they can empty the bins. As they do, I start on the paperwork. It is time to clear as much of the paperwork as I can before going home.

There are ninety-eight results waiting for me and after ordering them into normal, abnormal and indeterminate again, I clear those away. After twenty minutes, I turn my attention to the electronic prescriptions waiting to be signed and get rid of those. Fifteen minutes later, I make a start on the tasks and clear as many of the queries from the receptionists, queries from the diabetic nurse, prescription requests and other tasks as I can.

At five to eight the cleaners knock on my door, "We're leaving now doctor, are you ready?"

No, I'm not ready yet, but I refuse to stay on my own in the surgery at night. Safety in numbers. I clear my desk, grab my things, switch off the computer and follow the cleaners outside. On my way I also grab the box of prescriptions requiring signatures, I can do that at home and bring them with me in the morning. The letters have not been actioned yet, but they will need to wait, I'm only human after all.

At eight I drive off after a quick call to Martin to let him know I am on my way. He insists I call when leaving so he can estimate when he needs to worry if I don't get home on time.

CHAPTER 13

Tuesday, 8:05 pm

On my way home, I go over the occurrences of the day. Once again I'm left wondering if I am a good enough doctor or if it would be better to just give up on this as a bad job. When there is yet another advert on the radio to entice people to contact some solicitor's firm over alleged medical negligence, I again notice fury rise in me. What do they think? That doctors are making mistakes on purpose? I really hate this 'Blame, claim, gain' culture that has emerged over the last few years. It makes our job even more stressful than it already is.

Still, next, a song starts playing and I sing along with it somewhat off-key in an attempt to reduce the tension a little. Soon the tension flows out of me a little and I can relax a little more before arriving back home. Martin has no need of a grumpy wife, he has his own stresses already.

By the time I arrive home, Martin is working off his own stresses on the PlayStation. First, I make my way over to him and put a kiss on his head, "Evening sweetheart, did you have a good day?" Martin mumbles something and concentrates on the game again.

The kids are already in bed and this makes me feel like a neglectful mother. Especially after all the complaints from patients today, my self-confidence is shaky. Would giving up the day job make me feel better? No, it would likely only make me more grumpy and a worse mother rather than a better one.

After the detour to the living room, I run upstairs and change into something more comfortable. Next, I head for the kitchen and start preparing our pasta. We have to eat after all. Even if it is half-past eight already, we should still eat.

While I stir the tomatoes, vegetables and prawns and the pasta boils, I remember my half-eaten sandwich and put it in the bin. There is no need for that one any longer. The food remains on a low heat and I get the prescriptions out to sign them. These are out of the way by the time our meal is ready and now I call Martin down for the meal.

* * *

Over tea, Martin catches my gaze, "Long day, huh?" Next, he takes another mouthful of pasta.

I nod, yes it certainly was. "There were over fifty ring-backs, nearly twenty extras and nothing I did was good enough. Just a normal day like any other." As I shrug my shoulders, I eat another mouthful of pasta, "When I got in this morning only five appointments were left for same-day booking. But, I'm home again at least. Didn't get all the work done though, it will need to wait till tomorrow."

Martin nods. Life is not much different where he works. The life of any GP partner.

We eat our meal and after putting our plates in the dishwasher, Martin makes his way upstairs, "I'll see you in a minute."

Once everything is put in the dishwasher and this has been turned on, I get the bin bag and take it to the wheelie bin, then put the wheelie bin at the curbside. It is bin day tomorrow. I return to the kitchen and put a new bin bag in, grab my bag and switch the light off. Phew, it has been a long day and I can't wait for my bed.

* * *

Now it is time to go upstairs and get ready for bed. Martin is already warming up the bed and not long after I join him in bed. Today has been a very long day. After ensuring the alarm is switched on, we say goodnight and it's time to go to sleep. Nine already, past my bedtime, but it could not be helped. Although I am tired, the occurrences of the day continue to plague me and I have difficulty falling asleep.

CHAPTER 14

Wednesday, 2:45 am

The pressure of not wanting to miss the alarm wakes me at a quarter to three this morning. Although there should still be an hour of sleep left before getting up, sleep does not come again and I watch the alarm clock as the minutes slowly tick towards a quarter to four. At half-past three, I decide enough is enough and I get up. I might as well get a head-start. As always, I take care not to disturb Martin, he still has a few hours left before he needs to get up.

The Fitbit buzzes while I get dressed and I silence it. Yes, the day has started again already.

*   *   *

And, of course, it's the same old, same old. The first job on the list is to clean the bathrooms and I get on with that as soon as I'm dressed. While I clean the bathrooms, I run through the day ahead in my mind. It is Wednesday today, and that means it should in principle be an easy day.

On Wednesday I only work in the morning and should finish at one in the afternoon. This gives me enough time to drive to school to pick Alex up when school finishes at half-past three. Even when school is over an hour away from work.

* * *

When I get downstairs, the usual routine of baking bread, cleaning the kitchen, unpacking the dishwasher and doing the ironing and folding of the laundry starts again. There is little to no deviation from the schedule and after an hour and a half, this job is finally behind me too. The kneading of the dough is also always a form of stress relief for me.

* * *

By a quarter past five, the lunches are packed, and the laundry is done. Now it's time to get the laptop out again. Last night I did not finish all the work before leaving and I hate leaving anything undone. Nothing should be left to the next day if possible, or I will already start behind schedule. Playing catch-up all day is not my idea of fun.

Overnight new results arrived, another ninety-eight

to work through. These are finally cleared by a quarter to six. Now, I turn my attention to the letters I had left untouched last night. Again, I started with the red-flagged ones; the ones requiring attention and action. There are quite a few of those and not all my own letters either. Dr P is still on holiday and I have been handed Dr P's load too. Then I clear the X-ray results and make a start with the yellow-flagged and non-urgent letters.

 At six Archie and Adam join me in the kitchen to eat breakfast, "Morning boys, did you sleep well?" Both boys grunt a little but don't give a proper answer. The day is still too young for proper conversations.

 After reading another few letters, but still having sixty-eight waiting for me in the inbox, it is ten past six and time to put the laptop away and get ready for work. The remainder will have to wait until I'm at work again.

* * *

 With the laptop shut down, back in its case and all bags packed, I rush upstairs. I place the bags at the front door, ready to take to work with me. As I move upstairs to get changed for the day ahead, I realise I have left the laundry basket in the kitchen and I rush back downstairs, grab it and return upstairs, picking up Martin's lunchbox on the way.

After changing, kissing Martin goodbye, "See you tonight, don't work too hard," and grabbing my bags, I'm on my way again to start the day's work.

CHAPTER 15

Wednesday, 6:45 am

On the way to work, the traffic slows on the motorway. Even though it's only a quarter to seven, there has already been an accident and one lane has been closed down.

Great!

Hopefully, this won't take as long as it did ten years ago. At that time I was stuck between two exits with no chance of changing the route for four hours. Obviously, I got to work very late, and the planned surgery should already have finished by the time I arrived. Fortunately, I had phoned the surgery hands-free to let them know I was stuck and no further patients were booked until I arrived at the surgery. There was only an hour left until I needed to leave to pick the kids up from nursery and school. That had been a wasted morning. Both for the surgery and for me.

Fortunately, it is not as bad this morning. However, instead of arriving at seven, I don't arrive until a quarter to eight and the gates are already open. Some receptionists have already arrived. After parking the car, I move to the backdoor, unlock it and get in. There goes my chance of catching up on my work.

* * *

Michelle is in reception today and I walk in briefly to greet her, "Morning, sorry I'm a little late. There was an accident on the motorway and I got stuck in the traffic for half an hour." I hand her the prescriptions I signed at home last night, "Here you go, I brought a present," and give her a little smile.

Michelle looks at me with a sad expression on her face, "Sorry Dr Ellen, I've just put another box of prescriptions on your desk. The box was still waiting in the office for you this morning."

"Don't worry. It can't be helped. I'll try to get these done as soon as possible." Then I continue to my room, switch on the computer and get ready for the day ahead. As it is already ten to eight by now, I might as well go upstairs to check if anything is waiting for me in the office now and have a bathroom break to get ready for the morning surgery.

* * *

Again, I return to my room after and start the

preparations for the day ahead. A few more of the letters waiting are completed, and I notice the complaint I received yesterday. I will need to make some time to answer that one as well today. Officially we may have two weeks to answer a complaint, but I always feel the sooner it is out of the way, the better. I absolutely hate receiving complaints. As a perfectionist, I always aim to do the best I can for all my patients. A complaint to me means I failed in doing that and the realisation hurts a lot. It makes me wonder if I will ever be good enough, or whether I never was good enough in the first place. Still, I must be to have gotten this far in my life.

After putting the complaint to the back of my mind for the moment, I return my attention to all other jobs still waiting for me. The letters, electronic prescriptions which were put in my inbox since this morning, tasks that were sent already. At least I'm not on call today and that is something to be thankful for.

* * *

As I glance at the bottom of the computer screen, I see it is already twenty past eight and I start signing the box of prescriptions while keeping an eye on the appointment screen. Nearly half-way through the box, I notice the first patient has arrived and I wonder if I

DIARY OF A FEMALE GP

should just quickly finish signing the prescriptions or start surgery early; it is only twenty-five past eight after all. Deciding to sign the last few prescriptions, I have a chance to hand them to the receptionist before I start surgery. Good. Now my desk is clear again.

* * *

Once the prescriptions are in the hands of the receptionist, I walk back to my room, take a sip from my already cold tea and call the first patient in. While I wait for the patient to arrive, I check the notes to get a clue as to the reason the patient might attend, check if any blood tests or reviews are outstanding and wait for the knock on the door which follows shortly after.

"Come in."

CHAPTER 16

Wednesday, 8:27 am

My first patient today is sixty-seven-year-old Philip, who I diagnosed with type two diabetes six months ago.

There are two main types of diabetes mellitus. Type one, where the patient no longer produces insulin and requires insulin injections and type two where the patient still produces insulin, but the body does not listen to it as it should. Type one diabetes is common in young people and type two diabetes is more common in people after the age of forty. However, nowadays there are more and more teenagers diagnosed with type two diabetes, a problem caused by obesity, which puts a patient at an increased risk of developing type two diabetes.

So far, Philip has controlled his diabetes with diet only, but his recent blood tests showed a deterioration in his diabetic control. From a reasonable control at 49 mmol/mol 3 months ago, his HbA1c (the control figure) has risen to 60 mmol/mol. Good diabetic control is very important for his long-term health outcomes and especially for reducing the risk of developing the complications of diabetes. A good HbA1c would be below 48, an acceptable one below 53 mmol/mol. It is time to discuss the next step in his management plan with Philip today.

As these discussions take more time than the standard ten-minute consultation, I am glad to see the girls have booked him a double appointment, twenty minutes.

"Morning doctor, you wanted to see me?"

After the initial greeting, I talk to him about his blood results, "I'm afraid your diabetic control has worsened a little. Any idea how this could have happened?"

Philip tells me he has been suffering from a muscle injury to his left leg and has been less active than he was before. Less exercise means less burning of the calories and an increase in the blood sugar levels. Even though this may be a factor, I'm not convinced this explains the deterioration in his control sufficiently, "That may have had a slight influence, is there anything else you think of which may have caused the worsened control?"

Reluctantly Philip admits that the lack of exercise has also led to sitting in his armchair more and boredom. A boredom Philip has filled with eating snacks. Not quite healthy snacks, but sweets, crisps and cakes. Philip is fully aware this is not the recommended diet for a diabetic and is adamant he will take control of this a little more after today. Another thing he reluctantly admits to is an increase in his weight over recent months. It is a well-known fact that good diabetic control is more difficult to achieve if weight is not optimal. Philip's weight is now back in the overweight range after an initial reduction to a healthy weight in the first three months following his diagnosis.

We discuss the options open to him. Yes, Philip will gradually increase his exercise levels and will reduce the number of snacks he eats, hopefully decreasing his weight again in the process. At the moment he does not feel like this will work very quickly and we agree to add medication to his treatment plan today too.

At this point, I also reiterate the information I gave Philip a few months ago. Although it is very important Philip does everything in his power to control his diabetes well, type two diabetes is a progressive disease. This means that even if he does everything absolutely right, his control will eventually worsen due to a gradual reduction in the insulin he produces over time. If a type two diabetic gets old enough, he will eventually also require insulin. Only in a few very rare cases is it possible for patients to return to a prediabetic stage after significant reductions in weight. These people will remain at a high risk of developing diabetes again at a later stage in their life.

After a quick check of the other blood tests, which show a good cholesterol level and good kidney and liver function tests, we agree to start Philip on metformin.

Although metformin is an old medication, it is still one of the mainstays of diabetic treatment nowadays. This medication makes the body more sensitive to the insulin it still produces and therefore helps to move the sugar into the cells where it works as fuel. This way it helps to reduce the sugar level with little to no risk of the sugar level dropping too low.

His blood pressure today is normal at 125/75 and after giving Philip the prescription and advising to start the medication slowly to avoid stomach problems and advising to repeat his blood tests in another three months, he leaves. A little limp is present as proof of his muscle injury when he leaves.

* * *

The second patient today is ten-year-old Olivia. She is currently on her way to school and has come with her grandma as mum is at work. "I think Olivia has conjunctivitis, doctor. Can you give her something for it?"

When I check Olivia's eyes, there is no discharge from her eyes, and the white of the eyes, the conjunctiva, looks clear and white. There is a little redness surrounding Olivia's eyes, and the skin appears a little dry.

"Actually, there is no sign of conjunctivitis at the moment. In that case, the white of the eye looks pinker and the eyes will be producing a pussy discharge. At the moment Olivia appears to have mild eczema around her eyes instead. You can either use a moisturiser for this, making sure not to get any of it in her eyes, or even a bit of vaseline."

After advising to return for a review if her symptoms don't improve or if they worsen, Olivia and grandma leave. With a bit of luck, Olivia will still get to school in time, it is only ten to nine.

* * *

The nine o'clock appointment has not arrived yet. Instead, I use the time to take care of some prescription requests in the task list and take them to reception after.

"Here are a few more prescriptions for you, Libby. Hot of the press."

While I am there, I notice the next patient has now

arrived and I call Lisa in.

* * *

Twenty-eight-year-old Lisa fell down the stairs in a shopping centre and broke her left lower leg a little over six weeks ago.

"How is your recovery?"

"Well, the plaster cast came off a few days ago, but it is still difficult to cover any longer distances. As long as I don't walk more than a few minutes, it's fine. But, if I go for my shopping it's still difficult and very painful."

"Do you feel you can go back to work again now? Remind me what you do for work again."

Lisa informs me she works as a warehouse-assistant and is keen to get back to work. Her job involves a lot of walking and that may be too much for now. She has spoken to the supervisor who advised Lisa to get a fit note to state she is fit for work with amended duties. The supervisor has promised to get Lisa a desk job for a few weeks if she gets a note.

After issuing the note for amended duties, Lisa leaves again, a smile on her face; she is looking forward to going back to work.

* * *

Nineteen-year-old Izzy is my next patient. At the moment I'm running five minutes ahead of schedule and I'm pleased with myself. Seeing Izzy takes some of that happiness away again.

Three months ago, Izzy was sexually assaulted on a night out with friends at university. She always was a happy girl prior to the assault, but now she is depressed with a lack of self-confidence and she suffers from severe flashbacks. Although Izzy receives counselling, her progress is slow and the flashbacks happen frequently. She finds it difficult to concentrate on her assignments and study and needs a note to support her in her request for an extension on her coursework.

Most of the consultation Izzy is in tears, going over the assault, the flashbacks and her fear of going out at night. Although her friends are supportive, she is still unable to go out and enjoy herself. Her head remains dipped, hands fidgeting on her lap and Izzy makes little to no eye contact. After writing the requested note, which unfortunately is not part of the normal NHS work and therefore carries a charge, Izzy leaves with the note after paying the required private sick note fee. To have to request a fee for these notes does not give me a good feeling. Not when the patient deserves to have our support, but rules are rules.

* * *

And then it is time for my fifth patient today already. The amount of time I was ahead, has now reduced and shattered and instead I'm running five minutes behind. Oh, well, you can't have it all I guess.

Twenty-seven-year-old Jenny comes in complaining of abdominal discomfort and bloating. She has gradually increased in weight over the last few months and denies any possibility of pregnancy, "I'm just getting fat, should stop eating rubbish."

When I ask her when her last period was Jenny informs me she has no idea, she has always been irregular and doesn't keep track. "They come when they come and that's just how things are."

After asking her to lay on the couch so I can examine her, I have a good feel of her stomach. It is quite large and, if I am to believe Jenny this is due to obesity. However, I'm fairly certain I can make out a baby inside. Even if it is not moving at the moment, I'm fairly sure I can distinguish the head, the body and the limbs. No chance of pregnancy? I'm definitely not convinced.

"Jenny, I believe you may be pregnant after all. Would you like me to check if I can find a heartbeat?"

Jenny's eyes shoot wide-open as does her mouth. Speech appears impossible, but she nods. Her mouth opens and closes as if she was a fish out of water.

I make my way to the cupboard and collect the Doppler. Hopefully, the battery is still working. After putting a bit of jelly on the probe, I place it where I expect the baby's heart to be, and..., indeed, there it is. A fast heartbeat can be heard.

"That is my heartbeat, though, isn't it doctor?" There is a hopeful glint in Jenny's eyes.

Not a lot of patients have a resting pulse of around one hundred and twenty a minute. I move the probe to where it picks up her heartbeat, "This is your heartbeat. Nice and slow." I move the probe to the baby's heartbeat again, "And this is the other heartbeat. Listen, it's faster."

"But..., but...," Jenny can't get her words out easily, "I can't be pregnant. This can't be true." Panic appears to have overtaken her.

Well, I'm afraid it's too late now. When I examined Jenny, it appeared like the womb reached to around thirty-six weeks already, there is no going back now.

"Jenny, I'm afraid you definitely are pregnant. And, before you ask, it is too late for a termination. I estimate you are about thirty-six weeks already and you will need to start preparing yourself. It won't be long until your family gets bigger."

Next, I arrange for an emergency referral to the

midwife. If my estimation is correct, she only has about four weeks left. Not a lot of time to get used to the idea of becoming a mother and preparing for it. Not quite the surprise you would expect on your visit to your GP. And Jenny definitely looks pretty shaken.

* * *

After dealing with Jenny and the emergency referral, I'm running ten minutes behind. The next patient is thirty-three-year-old Michelle, who has always had heavy periods. Although there has been no change in her symptoms, she is now getting fed up of having to wear a pad as well as a tampon and change every half an hour to an hour. She also passes some clots.

When we go over some options and any reasons why she could not have any medication to help her with her symptoms, I explain there are two main options open to her. The first would be to go on the combined pill, which generally reduces the blood loss.

Michelle shakes her head, "No, I don't think that is really an option, James and I are trying for a baby."

The other option would be to try a different medication, mefenamic acid, which reduces the clots and therefore the bleeding as well as the period pain. Michelle would however not be able to use this when pregnant, but she should have no periods then, anyway.

With an agreement reached and a prescription in hand, Michelle leaves, promising to return if she still has any problems with her periods or has trouble tolerating the medication.

* * *

Now, it is time for the seventh patient this morning. Sixty-eight-year-old Jim has difficulty with his breathing, a cough, and brings up green phlegm. Jim has COPD, chronic obstructive pulmonary disease, but has no temperature at the moment.

"How is your breathing compared to normal?"

"Well...," he takes a breath, "it is...," then takes another breath, "a bit worse."

Jim's wheezing can be heard even without the stethoscope. His lips are red and his cheeks flushed.

On examination, there are crackles on the right side of his chest and his oxygen levels are 93%, reassuring me that at the moment Jim does not need admission. However, Jim will need antibiotics for his chest infection and after advising him to seek medical attention if his symptoms don't improve or if they worsen, Jim leaves, "Thanks, ... doc." I can hear him slowly make his way back to the waiting area.

* * *

At ten to ten, we usually have a ten-minute break booked in. This allows us to catch up if we are running behind or to look after personal needs if needed. As I am running ten minutes behind, today the break will be used to catch up.

My eighth patient of the morning is fifty-seven-year-old Felicity, who consults me with chest pains.

"Over the last month I have had these chest pains, they are right here," Felicity places her fist over the centre of her chest, "and they come on when I'm climbing a hill or running to catch the bus. I thought I should see you about this."

Felicity is right, she should consult us about this problem.

"What does the pain feel like?"

"Well, it is like someone places a heavy weight on my chest and then squeezes it. It is difficult to catch my breath."

When I ask whether the pain goes anywhere, Felicity admits it spreads into her left arm and sometimes into her neck and jaw. The pain only lasts for a few minutes if she rests, "So it can't be anything serious, can it?" and only happens when she does anything strenuous. After she tells me there is a history of heart disease in her family, the diagnosis of angina appears to be even more likely.

"These complaints seem to point towards possible angina. What we need to do now is the following. First, we need to check a few things, your blood pressure, arrange a few blood tests and arrange a baseline ECG. That is a reading of your heart." I fill the request forms as I speak to Felicity, "Although it is unlikely the ECG will tell us anything, it is still something we need to start with. Once we have the results, we can complete a referral to the chest pain clinic. They will arrange some further tests to find out if you indeed suffer from angina or not."

Felicity sits across from me and nods, "That's what happened to my brother a few years ago too."

"In the meantime, I'll give you a spray for under the tongue to try. If you find yourself in a situation where the pain does not disappear as quickly, you put one spray under the tongue. If it still doesn't clear within ten minutes, you will need to call for an ambulance to exclude a heart attack." With my gaze on Felicity to ensure she realises the importance but is not too alarmed, I add, "Chances are you won't need to do that, but if it does happen, you need to phone 999. Please come back after the tests for a review."

Felicity nods, "Thank you, doctor, my husband told me I should come to you. I guess he was right."

She leaves to go to reception to book her appointments, request slip and prescription in hand.

Sending a task to myself to keep an eye out for the results, I turn my attention to the appointment screen.

* * *

With my hand already placed over the button to buzz for the next patient, I notice an instant message pop up from our nurse Ruth, "Can you pop into my room for a moment, please? Dr K is on an urgent visit."

Just when I thought I had caught up. I log off from the clinical system to avoid anyone gains access to medical information who should not. There is no telling who would inadvertently amble into my room and read patients' medical notes, either on purpose or by accident. I knock on the door and enter the nurse's room, "Morning. You wanted me to have a look at something?"

Ruth nods, "Lily is eighty-seven, and we have treated her for a leg ulcer for the last month. Initially, it seemed to improve. Today it looks a little red and angry and I wonder if it is now infected."

There is obvious debris in the wound, swelling and redness surrounding it and a smell emerges as well. Yes, this indeed appears to be infected. After advising Ruth to take some swabs, I move to her computer and prepare a prescription for antibiotics for Lily. Fortunately, she has no allergies, which makes life easier. Ruth will see Lily for review in a few days and can keep an eye on the ulcer for us.

* * *

The toilet is next to Ruth's room and I make a pit stop while I have a chance. Then it is time to get back to my room, log back onto the clinical system and call for my next patient. If I ever thought not being on call would be an easy ride, I now know better. Anything can happen, even when you are not on call.

* * *

By now I'm nearly ten minutes behind schedule again. Sixty-six-year-old Violet has come with a rash on her chest.

"When did you first notice this rash, Violet?"

"Well doctor, the rash has been present for the last two days. One or two days before then, the skin started to itch and burn there, but I couldn't see anything. I first discovered the rash two days ago when I tried to scratch and it appeared a little bubbly."

"Does it still itch?"

Violet nods, "Yes, and when I try to touch it, hot

needles appear to shoot through it."

When I look at the rash, it covers the right side of her chest in a narrow line around her body from the back to the front. Little blisters lie on red skin and I am convinced Violet has shingles.

After explaining to Violet that she suffers from shingles, a viral infection, which can cause chickenpox in people susceptible to this, I give her some further information, "Shingles is caused by the same virus as chickenpox. When a person has had chickenpox, the chickenpox virus can retreat into a nerve root and reactivate at a later stage when the immunity is a little lower. This then manifests itself as shingles, as it has with you."

The fact that Violet has sought attention within three days of the rash appearing is good news. Especially in those over sixty, the pain from shingles can persist after the shingles disappears. Treating shingles with antiviral medication within the first three days of the rash appearing may not cure the infection or even shorten the duration, but it does help to reduce the risk of the pain persisting after it has healed. I explain this to Violet and hand her a prescription, advising her to take pain relief if needed and if this is insufficient, to contact or see us about this.

* * *

Fortunately, I have caught up a little and I am only running five minutes behind when seven-year-old Sam comes in with his mum and grandma, "It's his bowels doctor."

Sam suffers from constipation. He can go five days without passing a motion and when he does it is very painful and he sits on the toilet for a long time. Lately, the problem has worsened and Sam is scared to go to the toilet, holding it in by force. This has led to problems with soiling his pants. At school, he refuses the use the toilet and this has not helped Sam either.

Now I need to find out some further details, "What is Sam's diet like? Does he eat plenty of fruits, vegetables and fibre? Does he drink enough?"

Grandma is shaking her head in the background and tutting away, while mum explains Sam does not eat many things, "Well, he only wants MacDonalds, KFC and pizza. I can't get him to eat vegetables and fruit, Sam simply throws them on the floor if I put them on his plate. If I give him a portion of our meal, he will only sit at the table with his arms crossed and his feet on the chair, glaring at us. He simply refuses to eat anything. So, after tea, I give him some biscuits and crisps. I mean, that's better than not eating at all, right?"

Grandma is still tutting in the background, "I told

you, Sarah, you need to be tougher with Sam. Biscuits and crisps are not food. He needs fruit and vegetables, real food. But will you listen?"

With a potential disaster looming in the room, I divert the attention by first examining Sam's stomach. Hopefully, by the time I have finished, I can give the appropriate dietary advice without causing worse problems between mum and grandma.

Other than an obviously full colon, this is the large bowel, on the left side of his stomach, the examination is normal. This confirms the constipation we already knew was present.

When I get back to my chair, I notice another instant message has popped up from the nurse, "Can you pop in for a moment again. Dr K still not back." This will have to wait until Sam has left again.

"Okay, there are a few things you can do to help Sam. And Sam, you can help as well. To help constipation, you need to make sure to have a diet with fruit, vegetables and fibre and sufficient fluids. Although this is not easy to achieve, you really need to encourage Sam to eat these. And you Sam, you really need to eat your veggies and fruit if you want your stomach to stop hurting, okay?"

Sam nods, but I know better than to assume he will listen to the advice given.

After also giving a prescription for lactulose, the three leave the room with advice to return if Sam's symptoms don't improve or if they worsen. I enter the details on the notes, log off and join the nurse.

* * *

By now it is twenty-five to eleven. Sixty-two-year-old Edwin has come to see Ruth in minor illness clinic with a cough and she is uncertain whether there are crackles on his left lung or whether it is clear. Ruth would, therefore, like me to have a listen too. Although not a lot of crackles are present, some are indeed, confirming a chest infection. After printing and signing the prescription and leaving Ruth to advise the patient further, I return to my room to continue my morning surgery.

* * *

The next patient is sixty-seven-year-old Victor, who is on hormone treatment for prostate cancer. Victor's prostate cancer is stable at the moment, but he wants to discuss his painful breasts with me.
On examination, he has enlargement of the breasts, also called gynaecomastia, which is a known side effect of the treatment he currently receives. They are also

tender to the touch.

After explaining the findings and symptoms to Victor, he is more reassured, and he agrees to discuss it further when he sees his consultant in two weeks.

* * *

The next thing scheduled on my list is the second ten-minute break of the morning. As I'm again running ten minutes behind, this is used to catch up and I buzz for the next patient. When we decided to put these two catch-up slots in our morning and afternoon surgery, this was a good idea. More often than not we are in desperate need of them.

Forty-five-year-old Amanda tells me about what she expects are menopausal symptoms, "Simon has sent me. I have been really moody lately, crying one moment, happy the next and argumentative at times. It must be menopause, right? Can't you give me some HRT to help me with this?"

So far, Amanda has not told me any symptoms to fit with menopause other than mood swings and I know I have to dig a little further, "What are your periods like?"

Amanda looks at me confused, "Uh..., normal. Why?"

"Are they any different from how they used to be, or still regular?"

Amanda nods, "Yes, they are still the same."

I explain that this does not fit with menopausal symptoms. During menopause, the periods stop or become rather irregular. Amanda also denies the presence of hot flushes and I am getting more convinced her symptoms are not due to menopause, "Is there any other reason you can think of why you would be having mood swings?"

"Simon and I have been experiencing some problems lately. He says it's because I'm moody and menopausal. That I'm always argumentative. At times he calls me all kind of names under the sun."

"And what do you think? Are the problems due to you or is there another reason?"

Amanda admits Simon can be verbally abusive, telling her she will never amount to anything, that she is stupid and everything she does is doomed to failure. She believes him and has given up on her plans to study for a degree at university. Simon has told Amanda staying at home and caring for their three children is much more suited to her abilities. "But sometimes I just can't accept that and want to do more with my life. Simon is probably right though. Most likely I would fail. Better not to try."

Inside I sense anger building and I push it down. There is no need to force my own hang-ups on others.

Still, I feel people should never settle for less than they want or give up on their dreams. They should keep dreaming and who knows, one day those dreams might come true.

"Do you really consider that to be true?" It is probably the safest way of establishing whether this is what Amanda wants and needs.

"No, I still want to try and that is what causes all these arguments. Simon telling me I can't do it and should not even try. But I really want to try. He has even threatened to cut my allowance if I don't give up on this stupid idea. But if he cuts my allowance, I won't be able to afford the shopping we need. And if I can't afford the shopping, the kids won't have enough to eat. I guess I have to give up on my dreams or it will harm my children and I can't do that."

By now I'm hearing alarm bells. How controlling is this man? Is Amanda at risk? Are the children at risk? After a few more questions, I am satisfied the children are not at risk, although the situation is hardly ideal. Amanda is not at risk either, other than of having her dreams taken away from her. After handing a leaflet about domestic abuse and the help available to people in those conditions, together with an offer of support if she needs it, Amanda leaves telling me she will think things over. Perhaps she will enroll into university after all.

I do hate it when people are bullied by their family or others. As a child, school mates bullied me too, so I know exactly how they feel.

* * *

And again I'm ten minutes behind. These psychologically charged consultations always take far over the scheduled ten minutes.

The next patient is three-year-old Ben, who attends with his mother. Mum is convinced Ben is autistic, "He never listens to me, always wants to have things his own way. That is a sure sign of autism, right?"

Not quite, but it is better not to antagonise mum.

"So tell me about Ben, about his development and the problems you encounter."

While mum tells me about how Ben does not do as she tells him and is always doing things his own way, I observe Ben from the corner of my eye. He is very interactive, makes good eye contact and continually tries to grab mum's attention. Mum does not respond to his attempts, other than to swipe his hands away and tell him to sit down and behave. She then continues to tell me all about how naughty and disobedient Ben is.

Ben is playing with a car and takes it over to me to

engage me in his play. No, definitely does not look like autism to me. He crawls onto my lap and immediately grabs for the mouse to play with the computer. "No Ben, I'm sorry but you can't play on this computer." He looks at me with sad eyes, gets off my lap and continues to play with his car. Although he tries to get mum to play with him, she does not react to him. Instead, she gets her phone to check on a text she just received.

I explain to mum that Ben has no characteristics of autism as he is too interactive and involves others in play to make that diagnosis likely.

She gazes at me for a moment and it seems like questions run through her mind. Mum sighs, "Well it must be ADHD then, he must be overactive."

Now I ask her some questions about his attention span. So far, I already have seen Ben playing with his car for a prolonged period of time. Mum confirms his attention span is considerable, Ben can play with the same toys for hours on end, he watches television for hours and from all descriptions does not appear overactive. Still mum is playing with her mobile throughout the consultation, not making eye contact often. She appears to be more interested in whatever is happening with that phone rather than her son.

Is this simply a problem with how she raises Ben?

Still, I should not come out and tell her my suspicions. There is no need to antagonise mum as this will not help Ben. While I get ready to advise mum about the Early Help Hub, a service run by the council and child psychological services, Ben climbs onto the bed. There is a risk he will hurt himself and when mum does not take action, continuing to play on her phone, I have to ask Ben to be careful not to hurt himself.

I get out the information about the Early Help Hub and hand it to mum, advising her they may be able to help as they are specialised in behavioural problems. So far, I have not observed any of those, other than mum's inattention and disinterest. Other than specialising in behavioural problems, they also have parenting classes and I suspect mum could benefit from those. I do not mention these though. The hub can offer those if appropriate. After advising mum to return if the problems don't improve, Ben and his mother leave.

* * *

After the difficult consultation with Ben and his mum, I'm running twenty minutes behind. I really don't know why people are insistent on getting a label for their normal child. Why their own ineptitude needs to be blamed on the child. Still, the next patient is waiting.

Next is eighteen-year-old Vanessa who attends with her boyfriend. They have been together for six months and would like to take the next step in their relationship. Nowadays it is not often to find these couples who wait to have sex, and it is refreshing. She would like to go on the pill and Brendan agrees with Vanessa. There are no reasons why she could not go onto the combined pill as she requests, she does not smoke, her blood pressure is normal and we continue to discuss how and when to take the pill, the interaction between antibiotics and the pill, what to do if she forgets one and that she is still covered by the pill even in the week she does not take the pill. (Over the years it has happened more than once for a request for the morning-after pill to be received because the person in question had sex in the break-week.)

With the advice to use condoms too for prevention of sexually transmitted diseases and a review with the nurse in three months' time, the couple leaves hand-in-hand.

* * *

Nearly twenty minutes late, at twenty-two to twelve, surgery should already have finished, but I still have two patients waiting.

The next patient is thirty-six-year-old Alison, who complains about a sore throat for two weeks. The glands in her neck are normal, she has no temperature, no cough and her throat appears absolutely normal. She has no other symptoms pointing towards a cold.

What could be behind Alison's symptoms? She is obese, and this makes me wonder if she perhaps suffers from heartburn.

Alison's expression is surprised, "Yes, but that has nothing to do with my sore throat now, does it?"

After explaining that in some cases the acid burns the back of the throat to cause a sore throat, Alison seems to be on board with the idea, "Now that you mention it, there sometimes is a burning sensation in the back of my throat."

As per usual in these cases, I run through the factors that worsen heartburn, "Heartburn is known to be worse if people smoke, if they drink alcohol, eat spicy food, are overweight and if they use certain painkillers like ibuprofen."

Alison looks shocked, "So, I guess I'm doing everything wrong then. I know I need to lose weight, I smoke, I have a curry at least once a week and I love a few cans of lager at night. For my headaches and joint pains, I use ibuprofen every other day."

We agree for Alison to try to address these factors and I give her a prescription to help with her symptoms. After advising her to return in a month to review her symptoms, or earlier if her symptoms worsen, the door closes behind her. Hopefully, the medication can be stopped as soon as Alison has worked on the factors behind her symptoms.

* * *

Finally! It's time for the last patient of the morning.

Fifty-nine-year-old Jill has been booked in for a double appointment today. She recently had a few blood tests as she complained of excessive tiredness. This had initially shown a raised sugar level, and this was repeated as a fasting glucose soon after. Again this was a little on the high side and we repeated it one more time as a fasting blood test with the HbA1c, the diabetic control figure, included in the test.

Together these confirmed the diagnosis of diabetes and Jill was here to discuss the results and the new diagnosis coming her way. Usually, our diabetic nurse would see patients for education about their diabetes rather than I, but she was due on holiday for the next two weeks, which would cause quite a delay in seeing the patient and we decided to book Jill in with me instead.

"The receptionist asked me to see you about my results. What is this all about? What is wrong?"

"Have a seat. You have had a few blood tests recently. Do you know what they were for?" It is always a good idea to check the patient's understanding of the problem first. Sometimes they know more than we expect and sometimes they realise far less than we expect.

Jill sits down and gazes at me, "Well, I wouldn't be here if I did now, would I?"

This is my cue to tell her about all the blood tests she has had so far and I start with all the normal ones, which did not tell us anything at all, then tell her about the important one for today.

"The reason we asked you to return for further blood tests was that your sugar levels were a little on the high side."

"What does that mean?"

"As the repeat blood tests confirmed a raised sugar level, this means you are a diabetic." I allow the news to sink in for a moment before asking whether she knows anything about diabetes and what she thinks this will mean for her.

"Well, isn't that when people need to inject themselves? I won't do any needles though, no way."

"You don't have to worry about that for now." I

continue with an explanation of the two forms of diabetes and that she has type two diabetes. Type two diabetes often can initially be controlled with diet only and we briefly discuss dietary advice, low fat, low sugar, no excessive salt, in other words, a basically healthy diet. Generally, I prefer to give patients a three-month period to try diet only. That is unless their symptoms are such or their diabetic control is that poor that immediate medication is required.

Jill is pleased to hear this, and that insulin is not required at this point in her life. While I make sure she gets as much information as she needs, I also ensure to not give her that much information that she won't be able to process it.

"So, do you have any questions for me at the moment?" We have already been talking for the last twenty minutes and after answering some of her questions, I hand her some information leaflets from Diabetes UK, to read through at her leisure at home. Next, I give her the handheld record, which tells her everything about the diabetic care we provide, details of doctor and nurse involved in her care, her recent blood results and the targets we will work towards and then I ask her to make an appointment for the second part of her education into her condition with the diabetic nurse when she is back from her holiday.

Jill is happy with all that has been discussed and knows she can always contact the nurse or myself if any questions would crop up about her diabetes.

* * *

Phew, it is ten past twelve, half an hour after my surgery should have finished, and I finally get a chance to use the bathroom again. I move upstairs and check the office, grab the box of prescriptions they have prepared for me, the mail and Libby asks about a ring-back which has just been received. A patient has phoned about a cough and pain in the chest on coughing for the last three days. Can this wait until Dr K is back from a visit? After quickly checking the details Libby has written down, it appears this can safely wait and I move to leave the office.

"Dr Ellen, can you have a listen at this tape, please? The locum has dictated a letter and I can't quite make out what he said."

When I listen to the tape, I understand what the secretary means, but with some difficulty, I'm able to work out the missing word and inform her what they are. Then, I continue to leave the office.

In my hands, I hold the box of prescriptions, the mail including a list from the pharmacist with a request to check if it is okay to change patients over to a more cost-efficient medication and some medical journals. Seeing the list reminds me of the complaint still waiting for an answer in my room. That is one of the priorities before I leave today.

As I pass the practice manager's room, she waves me in, "Another busy morning?"

After confirming this, she tells me about her son who is currently on holiday in Tunisia. He phoned her last night because his bag was stolen, which had all his money in and his passport. Angela is understandably concerned and stressed about the situation, although he has reassured her he is fine. My eyes keep returning to the clock which shows it is half-past twelve already. I really need to get back downstairs and start on the paperwork, or I will never be able to get to school in time. However, I stay for a while longer to allow Angela to get this off her chest.

CHAPTER 17

Wednesday, 12:30 pm

When I return to my room around half-past twelve, I find someone has added a ring-back to my appointment screen. Huh? How can that be? I'm not on call today and, in principle, I should not get any ring-backs.

After opening the patient's notes, I find this definitely is a problem for the duty doctor and not for me. It's not an urgent problem either, so it can wait until Dr K returns from visits. Trish has put the ring-back on and I send her an instant message, "Is there any reason you put a ring-back on my appointment screen?"

While I wait for Trish's reply, I sign prescriptions.

Seconds later her reply pops up, "You're duty doctor today, aren't you?"

After informing her Dr K is today's duty doctor, Trish sends a message to apologise for her error and to inform me she will change the ring-back to Dr K's screen instead.

* * *

Now, I continue with the electronic prescriptions, signing them and signing a few of the prescriptions in the box I brought down with me too. Once the electronic prescriptions have been done, I move on to the tasks but notice there is another patient waiting to be assessed on my screen.

In the bottom of the screen on the clinical system, several coloured squares show, which contain numbers. Some are for the results, showing how many results there are in total, how many there are for me and how many there are with no clinician assigned.

Next to these boxes it shows the letters in much the same way, the total number of letters with next to it the number of letters assigned to me.

The next line of coloured squares shows all my appointments for the current session, the number of patients seen, the number of patients awaited, the number of patients who have arrived and the number of patients waiting for me.

The following squares show the total number of electronic prescriptions, and the number assigned to me specifically.

* * *

On the right side of the screen, the last row of squares indicate the number of tasks in much the same way. This way it is relatively easy to monitor the workload. Again, the group of squares relates to the number of tasks, total number, tasks assigned to the group I belong to and tasks assigned to me.

In the square of patients awaited, there now shows a number one. Another patient has been added to my list. As I don't want any patients to slip through the net through either my own or someone else's mistake, I return to the appointment screen and find another ring-back waiting on my screen. Why did no one alert me? Or is this again a ring-back added in error?

When I open the patient's notes and check details of the ring-back, it only states "Personal problem. Patient wants to speak to you."

Oh, yes, it is Eleanor, a forty-nine-year-old lady who only wants to see and speak to me. For some unknown reason, she only trusts me. We have patients like that, and I suspect there are patients like that in every GP practice. Usually, she wants to talk about her panic attacks and I take a deep breath and phone Eleanor.

"Oh, thank you for phoning back, doctor. I would like to make an appointment to see you, please."

Huh? Why did she not ask the receptionist for an appointment?

"Is there any reason why you wanted to speak to me today other than to book an appointment?"

"No there isn't. Do you have any appointments next week, perhaps?"

"Eleanor, there is no need for you to speak to me to book an appointment. Perhaps you can phone our receptionists to book an appointment?"

She agrees, and we finish the call. My mind boggles at why she would want to speak to me to book an appointment. Five wasted minutes in which more of the paperwork could have been completed.

* * *

Now, it is time to clear my tasks. I start with the forty-eight prescription request tasks and check each one to ensure they are appropriate. There are a few requests from mums for paracetamol liquid for their little ones, just to have in the cupboard in case of temperature or pain. Sorry, this is inappropriate, this is not part of what the NHS is for. I return those tasks to the receptionists asking them to contact mum and advise her to buy the paracetamol over the counter at the supermarket or pharmacy.

Recently, NHS England has also released guidance on self-care. This guidance states doctors should no longer prescribe medication readily available over the counter. These items include common moisturiser creams, hay fever medication, paracetamol and ibuprofen, gaviscon for indigestion, and a lot of other things like dry eyes eye drops.

Several of the prescription requests are for dressings from the district nurse or from a nursing home. Others are for a repeat of medication prescribed earlier, which the patients found helpful. I issue those that are appropriate for re-prescribing and send a task back to advise the patient to come in for a review of the medication. During that review these medications can also be added to the repeat list if appropriate, saving the patient, the receptionists, and us, time in the long run.

There are a few requests for a repeat of antibiotics. Only in a few exceptional cases, these requests are appropriate. In general, I return these requests to the receptionist with the advice for the patient to book an appointment at the surgery for a review and assessment for the need of antibiotics.

A few of the requests are appropriate and were appropriate for some time. I wonder why they have not yet been added to the repeat list and remedy this.

Next on the list are seven sick note requests. All seven patients are on long-term sick leave and require an extension of their sick notes. I check on each of their medical notes and they were all seen for a review in recent weeks and therefore can have their note issued without the need to be seen again first. One of these patients probably should attend a review appointment before the next note is due. I return all tasks to the receptionists to inform them the notes are ready and will be available at reception, adding the need for review before the next note is due to the one mentioned earlier.

One already. The next group of tasks to complete is the group of twenty-two requests for reauthorisation of repeat prescriptions. All long-term prescriptions should be reviewed at least once a year. I can review some based on the notes, others require the patient to attend the surgery for blood tests, review of chronic conditions or face-to-face reviews with a doctor. For each of these tasks, which usually covers several items at the same time, I check when their annual review for any chronic illness is due, send a task to recall these patients if they were not requested to attend for the review yet, and check if blood tests, blood pressure checks and a few other things are up to date. If everything is up to date, but the reauthorisation has slipped through the net, I reauthorise the medication to when the next annual check is due.

If reauthorisation of the medication on the list does

not take place, this means the receptionist is unable to issue the prescription from the repeat list when the patient requests the item, causing a possibly unnecessary delay for the patient.

Now it is time for the miscellaneous tasks. These cover anything that is not covered by the above. Any queries from the receptionists about a patient. Thirty-four miscellaneous tasks are waiting for me. Five are from patients concerned about the scare in the news with regards to the rise in blood sugar levels on cholesterol tablets. Should the patient continue to take the medication or is it better to stop them? I should probably phone them and speak to them about it as it would be unfair to use the receptionists as go-between and pass a message on they would potentially not fully understand themselves. I leave those tasks to the side to phone the patients later. Five tasks have been sent by Michelle about diabetic patients who have not attended their booked diabetic reviews, should she send another letter? Yes, this would be wise. We have the standard invitation letter sent at the first call. If the patient does not attend, we send out another, slightly stronger worded, letter. A third letter will be sent after this one with even stronger wording. If the patient still does not attend after the third invitation, a fourth letter is sent which spells out the risk the patient is taking by not attending. A note is added to the patient's notes to alert us to the fact the patient has not attended this year, we check the medication to ensure it is safe to continue these without the check, then change the recall date to the next year in the hope the patient will attend then. Another seven are relating to blood tests. On the basis of blood tests a patient has been invited to discuss the results, but they request the doctor to ring them instead as they wish to avoid taking time off work. I quickly check the results and find some results were actioned by my colleagues, but could easily have been given over the phone instead. I sent some of the tasks back with an explanation of the results and when to repeat the blood test. Now, I still have another three which need to be phoned with the results and I put them to the side for now, I will ring those when ringing those other patients.

* * *

As I check the time, I notice it is already a quarter past one and I will need to hurry if I want to finish all the work that needs doing. Time to ring the first patient regarding the sugar levels and the cholesterol tablets.

After confirming I have the correct patient on the line, I ask what the problem is. "Well, I'm worried after I saw the news this week. They talked about how cholesterol tablets increase the risk of diabetes. I don't want to become diabetic and would like to stop the cholesterol tablets. Can I stop them please?"

I take a deep breath, "Although it is your choice whether to take the tablets or stop taking them, I would advise you not to stop them. What you have heard in the news is correct, however, the risk is tiny and is far less than the risk you would run of having a heart attack or stroke if you were to stop taking the cholesterol tablet. So, what would you like to do? Would you like to continue taking the tablets or would you prefer to stop taking them?"

The patient is rather angry about how the news failed to mention that, and I have to agree with him. In view of the information given, he decides to continue with the medication.

Another four ring-backs follow along the same lines.

Now it is time to address the three ring-backs due to the blood results. The first patient is Melanie, who wants to know about her diabetic control levels. Dr P checked the results last week and asked for her to make an appointment with a doctor to discuss the results. What is wrong?

When I check her results, they are still not in the well-controlled range and a change in medication may be in order. Melanie is not due to book a review with the diabetic nurse at the moment, and any adjustments would come after seeing or discussing with the doctor instead. After discussing everything we would normally have discussed face-to-face over the phone, we agree to increase her diabetic medication slightly and to repeat the blood test in three months. Melanie will keep a close eye on her sugar levels to ensure they don't drop too low and contact us if she experiences any problems and she will arrange a repeat blood test in three months' time to monitor the effect of the added medication.

Next is Robert, who had his cholesterol checked as part of an annual blood test at his request. The cholesterol is 5.2 and my colleague advised inviting him to discuss this further. When I check his notes, I notice he discussed this with a doctor three months ago, including whether he would or would not benefit from a cholesterol tablet. At that time Robert was adamant he did not want to take tablets, and they agreed to check again after three months of adjusting his diet. His previous cholesterol was 5.8, and this means he has improved his cholesterol significantly.

Again I explain about his cholesterol level and compliment him on the achieved improvement. He still is not keen to start medication and we agree he will continue with the dietary changes made and repeat his cholesterol in six months.

The last ring-back is for Shirley, a ninety-one-year-old lady who was asked to see the doctor about her kidney function test. When I check the results and her notes, I notice there has been no change in her kidney function results for a few years, they are very stable. Shirley is known with chronic kidney disease stage three and has been seen about this a few years ago when the problem was fully explained to her. Basically, her problem is one of wear and tear of the kidneys due to the ageing of the kidneys. At least it is in her case. As there has been no real change, it is unlikely that this will become a problem for Shirley and I am unsure as to why my colleague wanted her to come to discuss her results. I guess the notes were not fully checked at the time due to the work pressure we are under continuously.

After picking up the phone, informing Shirley of the results and ensuring she still understands what the problem is, I have finally finished with the task list for now.

* * *

Half-past one. The next job is processing the letters waiting to be read and dealt with. The red flag ones first as normal, the yellow ones I can always read at home or later.

Some red-flagged letters contain medication changes made by the consultant. One of those is a change to medication GPs are not supposed to prescribe, but the consultant has requested us to take over prescribing. Instead of doing as I am told, I keep to the advice given by the powers that be and send the consultant a letter to request him to continue prescribing the medication if he feels this is appropriate. The only thing I change on the patient's notes is to put a note on as to my reasoning for the decision and also to put it on as hospital prescribed medication. In that case, it will at least alert us if there are any interactions with other medications.

By now it is a quarter to two and I leave the yellow flagged letters till later.

* * *

Now, I turn my attention to the notifications, the internal e-mails. There are a few requests for private sick notes in here and I add them to my task list. This is where the receptionists should have put them in the first place, as they would then immediately link to the patients' notes. I answer the notifications and ask them to do this via tasks in the future. As this is a recurring problem with the specific member of the team, I can't help but feel a little annoyed.

There are another few requests for ring-backs from patients relating to the cholesterol tablet scare and realising it is already five to two, I know I will need to get a move on. Today I need to leave before half-past two if I want to get to school in time. With a burning face and heart pounding, I keep an eye on the time and add the ring-backs to tomorrow's appointment list, noticing I will be on call again in the morning.

There is a knock on the door and Trish enters, "Can you sign these prescriptions, please? The patient has come to collect them and Dr K is still on visits." I sign them, realising objecting is only more of an effort than putting a few squiggly lines on paper.

There is a notification from the practice manager reminding me of the partners' meeting tomorrow and to ask if I have any items for discussion. I send the items I thought of and her notification also reminds me of the complaint I still need to answer, and my chest tightens a little.

* * *

Two already, not much time left to deal with the mail and the complaint. First, I look through the mail, separating important from junk mail. There is a special filing system for the junk mail and it is called the bin.

Nearly half of the mail ends up there. However much a pharmaceutical industry may wish me to prescribe their medications, I am not swayed by their glossy leaflets and factsheets. Instead, I prefer to act on evidence and cost-effectiveness. The advice the local medicines committee gives us is also invaluable.

Some letters in the mail are from consultants about our patients, and these should have gone to scanning first. I put them to the side to take them to the file room with me later.

There are four requests for medical reports. One from an employer, but no signed consent from the patient accompanies the request, and I put a note on the envelope to contact the employer and request this first. Another one is from the DVLA requesting information about a patient's epilepsy before renewing his driving license. The other two are from an insurance company as the patient has requested life insurance, both include signed consent from the patient. On the envelopes, I request the patient's medical notes to enable me to complete the reports after adding the date of the request and the date of receipt for my benefit on the envelopes. All will go to the file room later, too.

Now it is five past two. Should I leave now and make sure I get to school in time? I am tempted, but decide to work on the complaint instead.

Writing a response to a complaint is always a tricky business. Although we should always apologise for the mistakes we make or things we have done wrong, we should also be careful not to take the blame for things that are not our fault. Much like when you are in a car accident, really. Again I read Darren's letter and am left feeling awful. Am I really such a horrible person?

After opening up Microsoft Word on my computer, I start by expressing how sorry I am to have upset him and how this was never my intention. Then I summarise the concerns and complaints he has brought forward and next I address them one by one, apologising where I can, without admitting I was rude. I still don't believe I was and the most I'm willing to apologise for is if he considered me to be rude and that I never intended to come across as such. Once I finish the letter, I read it through once more, print and sign it and shut down the computer. By now it is twenty-three past two and I will need to rush.

CHAPTER 18

Wednesday, 2:25 pm

First, I get my bags ready. After grabbing the letters, prescriptions and report requests, I rush to the file room and hand them to the file room assistant. Then I continue to the stairs with the response to the complaint still in my hand, knock on the practice manager's door and hand it to her, "Afternoon Angela. I just completed the response to the complaint. Can you contact the defence union for their opinion and advice so we can get this sorted as soon as possible? Sorry, I don't have much time, I really need to leave to pick my son up."

Angela nods, "No problem, Dr Ellen. I'll get that sorted for you. Just drive careful. Enjoy the rest of your day."

I return downstairs, get my bags and leave. The rest of my day will only last a few more hours. It's nearly half-past two already when I should have finished my working day at one.

On the drive to school, I try to relax a little and push

the pressure from work back down again. My skin still tingles and thoughts of how I might not be good enough continue to plague me. Forcefully, I push those thoughts down. After all, I would not have made it this far in life if I really wasn't good enough.

Once I get off the motorway and drive towards the school, the traffic becomes rather slow, and the pressure builds up again. Will I get to school in time? It is ten past three now and school finishes at half-past. Depending on how the traffic behaves, I may be late. Parking will definitely be tricky today.

Once I get past the roundabout, traffic is not as slow. At twenty past three, I reach the parking lot and park the car. I grab the box of prescriptions and sign those before heading for the playground around twenty-five past three.

While I wait, I speak with Emily, the mother of one of Alex's friends. She asks about my day at work and I tell her it has been a little busy. Soon Alex runs over to me, "Can George come home for tea today? Please?"

Do I have enough food in the house to accommodate one extra? Of course there is, and of course, George can come with us. Emily turns towards her son, "You be good for Alex's mum, okay?" She bends over to kiss George on his cheek.

"Mu-um," George wipes his cheek, "Don't do that,

you're embarrassing me."

"Around seven okay?" Emily asks after turning towards me with a smile still brightening her face. Seven sounds fine to me for pick up time and we stroll towards the car. After getting the boys in the car, I drive home, the boys chatting excitedly about what they'll do when we get home.

* * *

Around four we get home. Alex puts his schoolbag down at the front door, ready for the next day, and the boys walk down to the kitchen after where I get them a drink and a biscuit. After putting down my bags, I return upstairs and change into something more comfortable. A deep sigh escapes as I realise the time for relaxing will need to wait as more work is waiting for me.

The boys have gone up to Alex's room to play, and I return to the kitchen and get the laptop out again. The non-urgent letters are still waiting for me as I did not have time to finish them before the school run.

When I open the clinical system, I find more results, letters and tasks have also arrived and even more prescription requests. No rest for the wicked, as they say, but I never realised I was that wicked.

I read the letters, process the results and the tasks.

After signing the electronic prescriptions, I put the laptop to the side and pull my personal laptop out. Time to check my personal e-mails and finalise the crafting blog-related things. As a way of relaxation, I make cards and I also run a personal and a challenge blog which needs updating at least weekly. E-mails related to this also arrive and need to be actioned.

Before I realise, it is a quarter to five and Archie, Amy and Adam return home from school. They also grab a drink and a snack and go to their rooms to relax or to do homework. While keeping an eye on the time, I go backwards and forwards between the two laptops, carrying out any further work that arrives while I can. The more work I get done now, the better it is in the morning. Coping with piles of work waiting for me is not my favourite way to start a working day. Or any day, for that matter.

* * *

At about twenty past five, I turn off the laptops and tidy them away. After getting flour from the cupboard under the stairs, milk from the fridge and sugar, cinnamon and eggs from the kitchen cupboard, I prepare a batter to make pancakes for everyone. The pancakes I make today are mini pancakes, called 'poffertjes' in Dutch, and we jokingly call them frying saucers. Eaten with icing sugar sprinkled over them, the kids generally enjoy them and the pancakes make a special treat when friends are over for tea.

When I have prepared the first batch, I put them in the oven to keep them warm and continue with the next load. The bowl slowly fills up and when I believe there are enough, I call everyone down for tea.

I reach the bottom of the stairs, "Teatime!"

Soon the kids are running down the stairs, stumbling at times. The scraping of the chairs on the kitchen floor and excited shouts, "Poffertjes! Yummy! Can I get some?" Before long, they are fighting over the last few.

While the kids eat, I continue to prepare more to keep a good supply going until the batter is gone.

"Oh, mum, there are none left! Archie took the last one, it's not fair!" Adam stamps his feet, "I only had three servings. Can't you make more?"

"Sorry boys, the batter is all gone. Another time. Who wants yoghurt?"

All kids nod their heads, "Me, me."

Now, I grab yoghurt from the fridge and add fresh strawberries from the garden; I quickly picked some while they ate the last pancakes. When their bowls have been licked clean, the kids return to their rooms to play or do homework.

* * *

Around six, I make preparations for our tea. After peeling the potatoes and putting them in water, seasoning the steaks and putting some petit pois in a pan with water, I wait until half-past before cooking tea. Martin will probably get home around seven and I like to have tea ready for him when he does.

Tonight the door opens around five to seven and I join him upstairs to warn him about the guest, "Evening, how was your day?"

Martin returns my hug, "Busy as usual. And yours?"

"Very busy as usual."

Martin changes his clothes.

"Alex has a friend over tonight. You might want to put something different on than your pyjamas."

When he nods, I return to the kitchen to make sure the food is okay. After Martin joins me downstairs, we sit at the table and eat our meal while discussing the day. As always, we do not share any identifiable details, patient confidentiality is important.

* * *

Emily texts at seven, "Sorry, ran into some car trouble. Will pick Alex up at half seven if that's okay."

The boys won't mind one bit, I'm sure. This mishap

gives them another half an hour to play.

"No problem, see you soon."

Martin looks up from his tea. There is a twinkle in his eyes, "Who are you flirting with now?"

After I show him the texts, and the plates are empty, Martin goes to the living room to relax, while I clear the kitchen and turn the dishwasher on. Soon after, I join Martin in the living room and read for a while.

At half-past seven, the doorbell rings and Emily picks George up, "Sorry I'm late. The car didn't want to start, and I had to wait for Tom to get home to use his car instead. Tom is looking at my car now to fix it; I'll need it again tomorrow."

"No problem, we could have brought him home if needed."

Then I turn towards the stairs, "George, your mum is here. Time to come down."

Dragging his feet, George slowly makes his way down the stairs, "But I don't want to go yet. Can I stay a little longer?"

"Yes mum, can't he stay over tonight?" Alex looks at me with hopeful eyes.

I shake my head, "No, not on a weekday. Maybe we can arrange something on a weekend. What do you think?"

Two heads come up and eyes twinkle, "Yes, can we?"

Then as an afterthought, "...please?" There is a hopeful glance on their faces.

Emily and I look at each other and nod, "Yes, we'll arrange that some time," Emily agrees.

The door opens and Emily and Alex make their way to the car. A wave and they're off.

Alex trots back upstairs to get ready for bed, and not long after I also say goodnight and go to bed. Another busy day will be ahead tomorrow.

CHAPTER 19

Thursday, 3:00 am

Last night was another restless one. I woke several times during the night with the feeling I had forgotten to do something but wasn't able to work out what this was. That sensation is still with me now. At three I wake again and I haven't been able to get back to sleep again since. Still, I remain in bed, hoping to catch a little sleep after all, and I do. Just before the Fitbit tells me it is time to get up, I fall asleep.

As soon as it buzzes, I get out of bed, leaving Martin asleep in a warm and cosy bed; I am so jealous of him. If only I could stay there too and cuddle up to him, but duty calls. In more ways than one; I remember I will be duty doctor in the morning today. After grabbing my bag, I sneak to the bathroom to get ready for the day ahead.

* * *

I dress and, although I don't fancy cleaning the

bathrooms today, start the task I've set myself. Today it is difficult to pull myself over that threshold. Still, if I don't clean the bathrooms, no one will. For a few months, I had a cleaner. The problem is that I'm too much of a perfectionist and someone else can never fully do the job to my standards. I also felt guilty for having someone else do a job I considered to be my duty.

The thought of having a stranger in the house on her or his own did not sit well with me either. Because of that, Mary would come to clean at a time I was at home. Instead of studying or doing something fun, I felt obligated to work alongside her. Or to even clean before Mary came.

"Hello? What is wrong with me?" Still, it was impossible to change and when she had to leave a few months later due to ill health, I decided it was better to just do the job myself again. And here I am at four in the morning on a weekday, cleaning the bathrooms. I've only got myself to blame. Looking back to my youth, my dad always maintained girls had to do all the housework. Indeed, I was expected to do the housework before I went to uni and cook as soon as I got home. Housework did not feature on his to-do list and, as my mum had a job too, he felt it was my job instead.

* * *

Cleaning the bathrooms never takes long, and I am pleased I completed the task. Now, I move to the kitchen for the other jobs waiting on an early morning, the bread-making, dishwasher unpacking, kitchen cleaning, laundry and ironing. After an hour and a half of doing these little jobs, they are also done, and it is time to continue with the next task on the list.

* * *

At half-past five, I switch on the work laptop and check the results received overnight. Again results fill up the inbox, eighty-six this morning, and these all need checking and processing; the work never stops.
 The fifteen normal results I soon file into the patients' notes, and then it's time to look at the abnormal ones. Fortunately, most of the abnormal results are not really abnormal, three are pregnancy results. An abnormal result according to the computer means the patient is pregnant. So, we can inform another three patients they are pregnant. I hope this is welcome news. Over the years we taught our receptionists to never start with congratulating the patient. Instead, we tell them to check the patient is happy the receptionists will relay the result and to only inform

the patient of the result if the patient is. In all other cases, we will contact the patient ourselves to inform them of the result. The approach I take is to ask the patient what result they are hoping for and then give her the result. Congratulations can then be offered to those who wished for this result and commiserations to those who wanted it to be a negative result.

Once I have cleared all the results, I check the tasks and complete those I had not yet processed yesterday, and those that arrived after I closed down the computer the night before. The receptionists have even added a few more electronic prescriptions, and I clear those too.

Next, I go to the unassigned tasks. This is a dump box where tasks arrive that were not assigned to any person or any group within our team yet. Often these are from other teams, the hospital and also prescriptions requested electronically by patients.

First, I check the online requested prescriptions and sign those as far as possible. Chances are they will end up in my inbox anyway, so I might as well get rid of those and open up some time for the receptionists to work on other important tasks. In the unassigned tasks, I also find a few tasks from a receptionist who accidentally has not assigned the task to anyone. I read the tasks and realise from the wording who they were intended for and assign them accordingly. That is, except for the prescription request ones. I don't know who they were meant for and complete them myself. Hopefully, my actions now will lighten my workload during the rest of today.

* * *

Before I know it, Archie and Adam come to get their breakfast, "Morning, did you sleep well?"

Archie answers me while Adam mumbles a little and bangs the cereal box on the table. He is not a morning person.

Six already, I work through the last few tasks, then close the laptop and go upstairs to get ready for work, "See you later, boys. Have a good day!"

Bringing the laundry and Martin's lunchbox upstairs with me as usual, I drop my bags at the front door and continue upstairs, tidying the laundry on the way. Some towels I place on the trolley in the main bathroom, clothes for Amy end up in front of her door. Martin's and my clothes and the towels for our bathroom make their way to our bedroom with the lunchbox.

Once I have changed, I move over to Martin to kiss him goodbye. He can still stay in bed for another half an hour. Now it's time for me to leave.

CHAPTER 20

Thursday, 6:30 am

Today's drive to work is uneventful. The traffic on the motorway is moving well and I listen to the radio, singing along with the songs. Although I love singing, I rarely do so in company. Insecurity and self-consciousness stop me from doing so. At seven, I drive up to the gate, get out of the car and unlock and open the gate before driving onto the parking lot and parking my car.

I enter the mileage on the mileage log and get out of the car. As usual, I grab my bags from the boot of the car, unlock the premises and enter, disarming the alarm on the way. Today is like every other working day so far.

* * *

At the moment it is still dark in the building and I switch the lights on in the hallway. Next, I unlock the door to reception and place the box with prescriptions

I signed while waiting for Alex yesterday afternoon on the reception desk. The receptionist will file those when she gets in later. Now, I continue my way to my room, unlock the door and place my bags in their safe place while switching on the computer. It is time to see the work waiting for me already. While I wait for the computer to start up, I get my cup out and pour tea from my thermos flask; it's important to keep fluid levels up. Over the years I have noticed horrible headaches will plague me if I do not drink enough. And an awful headache is not conducive to concentrating and performing the job to my best ability.

* * *

Soon the clinical system is up and running. When I check the notifications, I find another one from the practice manager about the meeting at lunchtime. On Thursday lunchtime there is a partners' meeting and we sometimes extend this for significant event meetings, clinical meetings, complaint meetings or financial meetings. Today we will also hold a significant event meeting, where we discuss anything that has happened which has impacted patient care, the safety of staff etc, even if someone prevented it before it occurred. The aim is to learn from mishaps and near-mishaps, to hopefully avoid them happening in the future. Most complaints fall under this umbrella as well and new significant diagnoses do too.

Angela wants to know if I know of any significant events which need discussing today or if there is anything I would like to add to the agenda. This is something to think about during the morning if I can. The most recent complaint somehow does not seem appropriate, although perhaps it should be. Darren could have turned nasty, and that would constitute a mishap. Especially for me. For the moment I put this thought to one side and continue with my work.

A few more prescriptions are waiting on my desk to be signed. The receptionist probably put the box on the desk after I left yesterday. I sign them and put them to the side to take to reception later.

Another ten online prescription requests arrived and I sign those. By now it is half-past seven and the sound of doors opening and closing reaches me. One or more of the receptionists have arrived to get everything ready for opening the surgery doors at eight.

With still half an hour before opening time, I decide I can check my work-related e-mails and open Internet Explorer to gain access to them. While I wait for the system to log me on, I open the appointment screen to check what is ahead of me already.

Not again!

Only five appointment slots remain unbooked for the entire day. Several of the appointments that should be available for same-day booking only are booked already and show a message next to it "Dr K request". Dr K likely requested these patients to attend today based on ring-backs, results or letters. As I feel rather annoyed by the fact they used so many appointments with this message, I open the notes to look at the reason the patients were requested to come today. The majority are resulting from ring-backs. And most of those appear to be non-urgent problems which could wait for a routine appointment rather than offering an appointment today and using most of the on-the-day-bookable appointments. Too late to change anything about this now, I will just need to get ready for another really busy day. At least we booked a locum for today, even if nearly all of his appointments have also been booked already. We really need to discuss this problem in our meeting again. This can't continue. I make a note to add it to the things I will ask Angela to put on the agenda.

A few of the appointments booked at Dr K's request yesterday appear urgent enough to need seeing today. But why weren't they seen yesterday already? Unless it was really busy, I would have seen them yesterday had I been the duty doctor at the time. Curious about how busy yesterday was, I open yesterday's appointment screen and find there were several ring-backs, but by no means did it appear unduly busy. Maybe there was an emergency eating up all Dr K's time. That is something I can't tell simply looking at the appointment screen. Well, I'll leave this for now, no use wasting time investigating when other work is waiting for me.

With a few minutes to spare before I need to get ready for the start of this morning's surgery, I check the e-mails and deal with those. Work-related e-mails are generally from the CCG (Clinical Commissioning Group, our local overseeing body) to tell us about new services we are supposed to provide. Sometimes this comes with extra funding, and sometimes they will expect us to do that as part of our normal contract with no further funding attached to it. Over the years our responsibilities and the things expected of us have gradually grown. Certain services which used to be provided in the hospital have now been moved to primary care and simply been added to our workload, as this is more convenient for the patient and to relieve the workload the hospital is under. Sometimes the services were moved as a cost saving measure. The hospital charges more for these services than the GPs get paid for them. That is, if payment follows those services. Although in principle I agree with making life better for patients, if it really does is sometimes open to discussion. If they pile too much work on the GP's shoulders, the quality of their work might suffer. There needs to be a good balance.

There is also an e-mail to announce local training for the coming week. On a monthly basis, we get together with other GPs and practice nurses in the area to receive ongoing training. In this job you never stop learning, things continuously change, more research is done, treatments develop and we need to keep abreast of all those changes. Next week will be an update on dermatology (skin diseases). After checking the details, I debate whether I should go to this one or whether I can do as much online. I have to pick Alex up on time after all, and these meetings take place on my afternoon off, Wednesday. If I want to go to the educational meeting, I will need to arrange after school care for Alex and there are a few problems involved with that. Alex does not like to go, and it brings extra costs with it too. If the meeting is not something I would benefit from, that means a waste of money and putting Alex through something he prefers to do without. I still have a few days to decide and leave the decision for later.

* * *

At a quarter to eight, the practice manager knocks on my door and enters, taking a seat, "Can I have a chat, please?"

Oh, no, what have I done now? Although I can't come up with anything I've done wrong, I'm not infallible, and it is possible I made an error or inadvertently upset yet another person. In response to Angela's question, I nod.

"Patricia came to see me yesterday."

No, I could not think of anything I did to upset our receptionist.

"She complained about a patient, and I wondered how we should deal with this. Apparently, Patrick marched up to reception yesterday afternoon and leaned over in a threatening manner. Patrick told her she was a good-for-nothing B*** and she should just do everyone a favour by running out and right in front of a truck. This started because Patricia could not give him a prescription yet, as it had not yet been signed. Although Dr K had received the box of prescriptions, he had not signed them yet. Patricia looked into it and found out Patrick requested the prescription late morning yesterday and Dr K received the box yesterday lunchtime. How should we deal with this?"

Why had Angela considered it important enough to discuss this with me now? This would easily have waited for discussion in our partners' meeting at lunchtime. Discussing it with all partners present, even if Dr P is on holiday at the moment, was preferable to only discussing it with me. One thing was certain though, Patrick's behaviour was unacceptable, and it was also not the first time he had displayed this behaviour. On two previous occasions we felt obliged to send Patrick a letter warning him his behaviour was unacceptable, and if he continued to display it, this would lead to removal from our list. The last time was about six months ago, and again he had fallen back into his old habits. I will suggest during our meeting we now remove Patrick from our practice list as mentioned in the last letter to him.

In an obvious place in reception, we display a notice that prescription requests take forty-eight hours to process, so expecting it to be ready within a matter of hours was unacceptable in itself. His behaviour following this was even worse. We will need to consider placing a barrier at reception to protect our receptionists. The girls (and guy) have a right to be safe at their place of work.

"Although I realise this is an important issue, I think we should discuss this at our meeting at lunchtime when Dr K is also here and can help us decide. It may be time for a removal letter, but let's see what Dr K says about it."

* * *

Angela agrees and leaves me to sign a few new electronic prescriptions. Next, I grab the box of prescriptions I already signed, and get up to leave my room.

At that moment there is another knock on the door and Michelle walks in, "Can I have a word?"

What now?

"I'm so sorry, Dr Ellen, but I have just received a call from Dr K. Dr K won't be in this morning as he is sick. We have a problem. All Dr K's appointments for this morning are already fully booked, what should we do?"

This indeed is a problem, the nightmare already starts before the first patient even enters my room.

"It can't be helped, we must do what we can and cope. If you girls try to rearrange the appointments you can, I'll see the ones you can't rearrange and those who turn up before you can reschedule them. Just fit them in where you can. We've done it before and managed; we'll do it again. I'm sure we can cope if we just work together like the great team we are."

Yes, I hope we will. Personally, I am not so sure, but I need to keep morale up. A lot of the practice rests on the receptionists' shoulders. Without those girls and boys, doctors would be nothing and could do nothing. In reality, it is not so much the doctors who keep the practice running as it is the receptionists. Well, we need the entire team. Together we can be strong and cope with the pressure placed on us unless that pressure becomes too much. Will it be too much today? Time will tell.

"But I'm so sorry for you, Dr Ellen, it seems like you always end up with these situations."

I'm sure that's not true, it must happen to my colleagues occasionally too. Although I don't call in sick often. In general, I will even get to the surgery if I need to hold myself up on the walls to make sure I don't fall down. I hate letting anyone down and will drag myself into work even if I don't feel well. Occasionally, I had patients tell me, "You don't look well, doctor. You should see a doctor." Which, of course, I do every day. Either at work or at home.

After I hand Michelle the prescriptions, I make my way upstairs to get ready for the nightmare that will be today.

* * *

A short bathroom break later, I return to the office and check the mail in my mailbox. The receptionists already look stressed, which is only to be expected.

"Morning, this is Libby from the surgery. I'm afraid Dr K has rung in sick and I wonder if we can reschedule your appointment," she makes some encouraging noises, "I understand, well, in that case, you'll just have to come over and wait until the duty doctor can fit you in. There will be a delay though as she will need to see her own patients as well as the ones from Dr K who can't be seen at another time."

Yes, that wasn't unexpected. Not everyone will agree to wait for a different appointment. The girls make noises towards me about how sorry they are for me, and I reassure them we'll be fine. We can do this as long as we work together as a team. When they appear to be a little less stressed, I make my way downstairs again and wait for the storm to start. With a burning face and a tense feeling in my chest, I enter my room and take a deep breath before looking at the appointment screen. Fingers crossed it won't be too bad. Even if I know that is an idle hope.

CHAPTER 21

Thursday, 8:05 am

When I look at my computer screen, I notice it is not too bad. At five past eight, only three ring-backs are visible on my appointment screen so far. It could have been a lot worse.

The first ring-back is from a mum worried about her three-year-old daughter, Emily, who has an earache. Mum would like her to see the doctor.

As the girls are busy enough already phoning patients to cancel appointments, I ring mum myself.

"Hi, is that Emily's mum?" After mum's confirmation, I ask her how long it will take mum and Emily to get to the surgery safely.

"We can be there in five minutes."

After I offer an appointment for Emily around ten past eight, I continue with the next ring-back.

* * *

The next person I speak to is the mum of five-year-old Aaron, who has suffered from a sore throat for the last two days. Mum would like him to be seen and when I check when they can get here, we agree on an appointment at twenty past eight. As my morning surgery starts at half-past eight, I can just squeeze them in front of my normal surgery.

Good, so far I'm still in control.

* * *

By now three-year-old Emily has arrived and I call them in.

Mum looks anxious and plays with Emily's hair, twisting the hair around her fingers lightly before letting the hair spring back again. "Emily started complaining of her right ear two days ago. It seemed to get better, but it is worse again today."

Mum bites her lips while I examine Emily. "Can I check your temperature with this?" I hold up the thermometer and Emily nods shyly.

When I check Emily's temperature, it is raised at 38.2 C. Again, I ask Emily's permission to examine her ears. The right eardrum is red and bulging, evidence of a middle ear infection. Unfortunately, Emily is allergic to penicillin and I have to give her a prescription for a different antibiotic, "Here you go. Some medicine to make your ear better. Can you carry that without it getting ripped?"

Emily nods her head and proudly takes the prescription, holding it close to her body to keep the prescription safe. A small smile plays on Mum's face, "Thank you, doctor."

Armed with the prescription and advice to return if her symptoms don't improve or worsen, they leave and it is time to continue with the next job on my list.

* * *

Sam has not arrived yet and I look at the next ring-back. Fifty-six-year-old David requests a cream for his skin condition. Unfortunately, he has not told the receptionist which cream he is after and I need to phone him to confirm this. He tells me he wants a repeat of the Diprobase, which usually works. After issuing the prescription and informing David he can collect the prescription from reception later today, I advise him to return for a review if the cream does not have the desired effect.

* * *

Five-year-old Sam has arrived now and another two ring-backs have joined the appointments on my appointment screen.

Just when I thought I was staying in control.

Sam enters the consultation room with his dad. The story is exactly as I was told on the phone. Two days of a sore throat and it is getting worse.

His temperature is raised at 38.7, Sam has a fever. The glands in his neck are enlarged, as are his tonsils, which also have white spots covering them. When I check his ears and chest, these are normal.

As always, I ask about any allergies to medication. We are here to make things better. Not worse than they are already.

"No, Sam has no allergies, doctor."

I issue a prescription for penicillin and ask them to return if he worsens or does not improve. Now it's time for the next job.

* * *

Checking a throat and issuing a prescription fortunately does not take much time and none of the booked patients have arrived yet. None of mine and none of Dr K's either. Instead, I turn my attention to the appointment screen, there are five ring-backs waiting for me.

Thirty-two-year-old Adam has injured his back while gardening and would like to book an appointment with a doctor today. As none are available, they passed the request to me.

After picking up the phone, I dial his number.

"Morning, this is Dr Ellen. I understand you want an appointment today. Will ten past ten suit you?"

"Do you not have any other times? I still need to get dressed."

"Sorry Adam, but this is actually a non-existing appointment which I created especially for you. This also means you will need to prepare yourself to waiting for a while as I may run late if there are any emergencies."

I continue to explain I am working through an excessive workload today because of the illness of one of my colleagues. At least Adam now knows what he is in for, and this will hopefully stop him complaining if he has to wait. Even prior to the explanation and the possible wait, he sounded grumpy enough already.

* * *

Now, I turn my attention to the fifth ring-back of the day. None of the patients on the appointment list arrived yet, and I make the best of the opportunity this gives me. The fifth ring-back is from seventy-six-year-old Edward.

"Morning Edward, what can I do for you?"

"Well, I have this cough," and he immediately coughs

and wheezes on the other end.

When I ask him if he is bringing up any phlegm, he confirms it is thick and green. This is a sign he may suffer from a chest infection, and I offer him a sit-and-wait appointment so I can listen to his chest and examine him. Edward accepts the appointment offered at twenty past ten and is aware there may be a wait. Usually, I would send a task to the receptionists to offer and book these appointments, but they have their hands full already with calling patients to cancel and reschedule appointments. We all need to help each other on days like these.

* * *

After I end the phone call, Dr K's first patient has arrived, but my own patients not yet. Desperate to keep as much control of things as I can, I call the first patient in.

Forty-five-year-old Melinda works as a receptionist and is unable to talk much. Her voice keeps coming and going, and it is difficult to understand her. This does not work very well with her job, and she, therefore, requests a sick note. She also has a chesty cough.

When I listen to Melinda's chest it is clear, "Good, your chest is fine at the moment. Unfortunately, there is no treatment available for a lost voice. Try not to whisper but to talk in as normal a voice as possible if you need to talk. Talk as little as you can."

"But I need to speak in my job," Melinda's voice is croaking and squeaking and disappears at times, "can't you give me a sick note?"

I explain to Melinda she does not require a sick note at this point in time. Melinda has so far not been off sick yet and she can put a self-certificate in for up to a week if needed. Only if the sickness period extends the week, does she need a note from her GP. And that is unlikely. Happy with the explanation and promising to return if she does not improve or if she gets worse, Melinda leaves.

* * *

It is now twenty-seven to nine and my first patient has also arrived. Fifty-two-year-old Angela suffers from breast cancer and has had surgery to remove the lump. The breast cancer was detected when she attended for routine breast screening three months ago.

"Morning Angela, how are you doing?"

Angela throws her shoulder-length brown hair over her shoulders, "Not bad at all. The wounds all healed very well and I can cope with the chemotherapy too."

Then she touches her hair again, "I'm not sure how long I'll still have this, though. The oncologist told me it's likely I'll lose my hair with the chemo. Still, it's better than leaving my teenage kids, right?"

I nod, "Yes, at least now you've got a good chance of being here to see them grow up." The letters from the specialist informed me they expected Angela to make a full recovery following the surgery, and the chemotherapy was only extra security to ensure it would not return. Of course, there are no guarantees in life, but the odds look good.

"As my immunity is reduced with the chemotherapy, they have advised me to stay off work another six weeks. Could you give me a fit note for that, please?"

I give Angela a note and offer her support if she needs it. Then she leaves and I need to continue with the next item waiting for me.

* * *

By now, Dr K's second patient has arrived. This is thirty-seven-year-old Dylan, who needs a review of his medication. Dylan started on an anti-depressant about four weeks ago and has now come to review his depression and the medication. This way we can make sure Dylan is improving and the medication works.

"Thanks, doctor, I'm feeling much better."

When I run through the depression questionnaire with Dylan again, this has improved, and he has no problems tolerating the medication. Just like the previous time Dylan attended the surgery, he denies any suicidal thoughts. After advising him to continue the medication, I give him another prescription, which now also is on his repeat list. Anti-depressants are usually continued for at least six months after the patient has improved to what their usual self is. Research shows the risk of a relapse of the depression is much reduced by taking this simple precaution.

Dylan has been able to work even with his depressive symptoms and he does, therefore, not need a sick note.

"Please return if your symptoms worsen or don't improve any further. Remember to continue the medication for at least six months. I would like you to return for a review in six months, even if you are doing well. Provided you are well then, we can consider reducing and stopping the medication again."

Dylan agrees and leaves. Now it is time for the next patient.

* * *

At seventeen to nine, it is time to see the second patient booked onto my list. Although fifty-six-year-old Thomas' appointment was due at twenty to nine,

I'm still not doing too badly considering the double workload. Several other ring-backs have also arrived and the sensation of losing control takes hold. I hate not being in control, but it is unavoidable. A tightness is building in my chest and I feel my face reddening.

Thomas wants to discuss his concerns about his cholesterol medication. As he has heard in the news, these can increase his sugar levels. As a diabetic, he wants to ensure his sugar levels are as good as possible and he does not want to risk the tablets worsening his control and leading to a need for more medication.

"What do you think, should I stop taking them?" There is a concerned look in his eyes.

After again explaining how the benefits of the tablets outweigh the potential risk of worsening his diabetes, he decides to keep taking his medication. Yes, this little scare has brought its own addition in workload as I already expected.

* * *

At ten to nine, I call in Dr K's third patient. My third patient has also arrived, but slightly later and with the double workload I have decided to see the patients on a first-come-first-serve basis.

Seventy-three-year-old Mabel is not impressed to see me, "I thought my appointment was with Dr K today.

If I had known it was with you instead, I would have rearranged the appointment."

Okay then, it is absolutely in her right to do so, "I'm really sorry about that. Dr K has called in sick this morning. If you wish, we can re-book your appointment with Dr K."

"No, no, I'm here now. Better get it over and done with," Mabel huffs. "My right knee has been playing up lately and I want something done about that. The painkillers are no longer doing anything for me."

Mabel is known with osteoarthritis (ageing of the joint) and is currently on co-codamol 8/500 (this is a combination of 8 mg codeine and 500 mg paracetamol). Although Mabel takes two tablets of this four times a day, her pain is not sufficiently under control, and she would like something stronger for the pain.

"Would you like to try co-codamol 30/500 instead? This is a little stronger than you are taking at the moment. Instead of 8 mg, it has 30 mg codeine in it."

Mabel's expression softens, and she no longer appears as displeased as she was when she first entered my room. The medication can, however, cause more constipation and drowsiness than the lower version does, and I advise her of this. After I also advise her not to drive if any drowsiness occurs and to return if she has problems tolerating the medication or the pain does not respond to the stronger dose, she leaves.

The current recommendation is not to use this type of medication long-term as it offers little in lasting benefits and has many side-effects. The medication also carries a potential risk of addiction, which we would like to avoid. A referral for physiotherapy may be more beneficial.

* * *

And now it is time for my third patient. Even more ring-backs have arrived and my expectations of this day becoming a nightmare look set to be fulfilled.

Eighty-four-year-old Minnie has come complaining of her right hip. This hip is causing her increasingly more trouble, and on maximum pain relief, she can only just manage. Walking is more of a problem than it has been, and she would like to find out if the time has come for her to request a hip replacement. If the pain and the osteoarthritis are interfering with her life this much, the time may very well have arrived and referral to the orthopaedic surgeons appears to be appropriate. But before we do, we need an up-to-date X-ray of her hip. After filling in the form, I hand it to her, asking her to see us for the results two weeks after she has had the X-ray done. At the local hospital, she can attend and wait for the X-ray to be done without an appointment.

* * *

Next on the list is the fourth patient on my appointment screen. No further patients for Dr K arrived so far, but several other patients believe they need an appointment with a doctor today and are waiting for me to ring them back about their medical concerns.

Nineteen-year-old Jack has come with a tickly cough, runny nose and blocked ears, "Can you get me some antibiotics, doc?"

After checking his chest, ears and throat and finding all in order, I explain his symptoms are caused by a cold virus. Cold viruses do not respond to antibiotics and these would, therefore, not be helpful for Jack's symptoms.

"But surely I must have an ear infection. Why else would my ears be blocked?"

As I turn towards Jack again, I wonder how I can explain the situation to him in the best way.

"Have you heard about the Eustachian tube?"

Jack has a confused look in his eyes.

"There is a little tube that runs from your middle ear to your throat. We call this the Eustachian tube. When this tube works well and is open, air fills the middle ear and your ear performs normally. During a cold, the lining of this tube swells and mucus gets trapped in the middle ear. When that happens, your ear seems to be blocked, and it can dampen your hearing. Sometimes it even appears like you are underwater. This is innocent but uncomfortable and you feel like your ear needs to pop."

Jack nods. He seems to follow the explanation so far. "So what can you do about that, doc?"

After I explain how steam inhalation can help with this and advise Jack to return if his symptoms don't improve or if they worsen, he leaves.

* * *

So far, no further patients have arrived and I take the chance to look at the sixth ring-back.

Twenty-seven-year-old Stephen believes he has an infected ingrowing toenail and would like someone to check this. Although this may not be as serious as he feels, I ring him and ask Stephen to come to the surgery around twenty past ten for a sit-and-wait appointment. In other words, he arrives, books in, sits in the waiting room and waits until I can examine his toe.

* * *

In the meantime, Dr K's fourth patient has arrived. Eighty-seven-year-old Thomas has problems with his waterworks he tells me, "It takes a while to get started if you know what I mean. Then when I get started, the stream is weak, and it takes a while to empty my bladder. After I finish, I need to wait for a few minutes, to make sure I really have finished or risk wetting myself. I wonder if it's my prostate."

That is what I wonder too, it certainly appears that way. To properly examine Thomas' symptoms, an internal examination of the back passage is needed and blood tests and a urine test need ordering. When I offer to examine him, Thomas asks if he can see a male doctor for that. Men often feel embarrassed to undergo this examination, and especially so if it is a woman performing the examination.

"No problem. In that case, we must book you in with Dr K when he returns to work. When you book an appointment with the nurse for the blood tests, you can ask the receptionist if any appointments are available for Dr K. You may need to book on the day, though."

The appointment system allows only a proportion of the appointments for booking in advance. Another few are available to book online, and the rest is available to book on the same day as the appointment. Unless Thomas wants to wait a few weeks for the appointment, it is likely he will need to book an appointment on the day.

I give him a form to arrange the blood and urine tests and a questionnaire to fill about his symptoms. Thomas should bring the filled questionnaire to his next appointment with him. He agrees with this solution and leaves.

* * *

My next patient is forty-eight-year-old Sandra who is irate to have been kept waiting, "You never run on time, do you?"

Come on, it wasn't that bad, was it? Her appointment was for ten past nine and it's only a quarter past nine now. In fact, I think I have done quite well considering. Still, arguing with a patient is never advisable, "I'm really sorry to be running late. Today it is out of my control, I'm afraid. Dr K called in sick today and I'm coping with Dr K's workload as well as mine and I am on call to top it all off."

Sandra huffs, "Okay, I'll allow it this once. Just do better next time." Her posture reminds me of a recalcitrant toddler, only a lot angrier.

The problem today is one of possible haemorrhoids or

piles. Sandra has noticed some lumps at her back passage which are itchy and sore, but she has had no bleeding from them. After she accepts the offer to examine her, piles are confirmed. The internal examination of her back passage does not reveal any abnormalities. With a prescription for some Anusol cream to ease Sandra's symptoms and the advice to return if her symptoms don't improve, she leaves. Hopefully, she is more satisfied now than when she first came in. Still, we can't satisfy everyone.

I dread to imagine what would happen now. Recent guidance advises GPs no longer prescribe Anusol as it is available to buy over the counter. Instead, doctors should advise the patient to buy the cream themselves. Sandra would likely explode in further angry and abusive words.

* * *

The sixth patient on my appointment list today is ninety-two-year-old Joseph, who attends with his daughter. Joseph suffers from Parkinson's Disease and, as is a common occurrence with this illness, often suffers from constipation.

"Dad would like to have another prescription for lactulose please."

Lactulose has always helped Joseph with this problem,

and I know of no reason why I can't get him another prescription for it. But why on earth did he come to the surgery to request a prescription? Joseph's mobility is very poor, and getting here costs him a lot of effort. They could just ask for a repeat prescription and we would likely issue it without a need to attend the surgery.

Joseph's daughter smiles, "Dad always enjoys visiting you and was adamant he wanted to come and see you today."

Although this makes me smile and a warm sensation blossoms in my chest as a result, I'm still sorry he took all this trouble to get a prescription. Joseph's warm smile makes the day seem brighter, and I soak it up to help me get through what promises to be a long and difficult day.

* * *

And now it is time for the fifth patient on Dr K's list. Fifty-five-year-old Kay was booked in for twenty past nine and it is now just past half-past nine. Kay is not happy the appointment today is with me, "The receptionist could have told me it was you. I don't really want to see you. Why is my appointment not with Dr K today? I asked for Dr K."

After I explain Dr K phoned in sick this morning and I

am therefore seeing Dr K's patients as well as my own, Kay shrugs, "Okay then. You'll have to do, I guess."

Lovely, here I am busting my gut to consult with all these patients and I 'will have to do'. What a downer after Joseph. When I ask Kay what I can do to help, she points to a mole on her right temple, "Can you look at this?"

On her right temple is a small nodule which is slightly shiny and it has all the hallmarks of what we call a basal cell carcinoma. This is one of the more benign forms of skin cancer and one that easily can be taken care of. After I explain this to her, I fill in a form for referral to the dermatology department, for an appointment within two weeks if at all possible. Kay accepts the form and will take this to reception to book an appointment for this.

I hope this will atone for the fact she was seeing me today and not Dr K.

* * *

Although it is twenty-two to ten already and my half-past nine appointment has arrived, the long list of ring-backs is nagging at me. I decide to first call the seventh ring-back before calling in my next patient. Logic tells me there is no difference whether I first make my way through the appointments and deal with the ring-backs second but keeping the ring-back list down gives me a sense of control. Still, one of the ring-backs could require urgent attention, even if the receptionist did not pick up on this. Receptionists have not received medical training and we can not expect them to triage patients unless we supply them with the appropriate training and support for this.

The mum of twelve-year-old Kimberley has phoned as she wants her daughter to be seen today due to her heavy periods. After offering a sit-and-wait appointment at half-past ten, I continue with the next patient. Getting into an argument over the urgency of the appointment is time I can't afford today, and it is easier to offer an appointment instead.

* * *

By now the next patient for Dr K has arrived too. Fifty-one-year-old Fiona is first in line to come in, though. I see her ten minutes late, at twenty to ten, and Fiona wants to have some help with her menopausal symptoms. Her last period was eight months ago, and a blood test has confirmed she is menopausal. Fiona's symptoms mainly consist of hot flushes, although she also has a few mood swings. As they do not cause her too much trouble, the hot flushes are the main reason for her request.

"I was wondering about HRT doctor, but there has been so much about it in the news in recent years. Can you tell me some more about it?"

Again it is time to go into explanation mode and talk about risks and benefits, something that forms a large part of my job. After explaining that HRT brings with it an increased risk of breast cancer, heart attacks and strokes, even if that risk is small, and informing her HRT works well for the hot flushes, but is not helpful for protecting against osteoporosis (brittle bones in the elderly) in the long term, Fiona prefers to persist without HRT for now. Fiona will come back if she changes her mind or the symptoms become too difficult to cope with.

* * *

Noticing even more ring-backs arrived while I helped Fiona with her problem and my next patient is now also waiting, the heat in my face rises. I take a sip from my now cold tea and call Dr K's next patient in.

Forty-seven-year-old Steven takes a double-take when he enters my room, "Huh? I thought I was seeing Dr K today."

After once more explaining Dr K is off sick today, Steven continues, "So, are you a locum?"

Uh, no, I've been here for over twelve years and even

longer than Dr K has been.

"How come I've never seen you then?"

To be honest, I don't know, unless it has something to do with the fact Dr K works full time and I am part-time.

Why doesn't Steven come to the point? I have more to do today, far more. When I ask him what I can do for him today, he tells me he has a rather embarrassing problem. That gives me a pointer, as in most cases where a patient tells me there is an embarrassing problem, this is a problem in their private area. Indeed, Steven also has a problem there. He has found a blemish on his penis and wants the doctor to have a look at this. Steven is happy for me to examine him, although I offer him to re-book with a male doctor instead and he shakes his head, "I'm here now, after all."

The blemish turns out to be an innocent birthmark, and I reassure Steven of this. He leaves a happy man, I guess he was more worried about it than he let on.

* * *

At two minutes to ten, I call the ten to ten patient in. Forty-eight-year-old Lesley comes to discuss her diabetic control. On the last blood test, we noticed a deterioration of her diabetic control from 48 to 56 and

Lesley had been asked to come to see me about this.

"Well, I've been eating all the wrong things lately and gained a lot of weight. I'm ashamed of myself, but the depression was much worse over recent months. I know I can do better than this and I would like you to give me some time to prove that before adding any further medication. Last week I've started the gym and I am already doing better with my mood and diet." Her eyes look at me pleadingly.

Lesley appears to have taken some good measures to help herself, and I praise her for this. Simple measures like a change in diet and exercise can make a significant change to a patient's diabetic control.

After agreeing to make the planned changes and repeat the blood tests after three months, she leaves looking confident and happy. Hopefully, she will be successful in her attempts. Even if the diabetic control refuses to return to acceptable levels, it will probably lead to a significant improvement.

* * *

Another patient for Dr K is waiting for me. It is ten past ten and my extra patients have not arrived yet. Several more ring-backs did arrive though. When I check Dr K's remaining list for this morning, I notice the girls cancelled most of the appointments. One is still on the list for twenty past eleven though.

Forty-three-year-old Martin requests a sick note for amended duties. He is recovering from an appendicectomy (surgery to remove his appendix) and this still hurts when he lifts things. As Martin does a lot of lifting at work, he needs a note for amended duties to allow him to not lift as much as normal. As this seems an appropriate request two weeks after surgery, I give him a note for two weeks of amended duties.

* * *

By now it is a quarter past ten and I am desperate to reduce the number of patients waiting for me to return their call. The enormous amount of waiting patients turns up the pressure and I need to gain control in some little way; I hate the sensation of losing control of my workload.

My first extra patient has arrived, but first I want to reduce the number of waiting ring-backs. The possibility that more extra patients lurk in the ring-back list is substantial and the sooner I get those added to the list, the better it is. Better at least than finding out more patients need adding to the list after I've seen the extra patients. That would mean a possible waste of time waiting for patients to arrive for their improvised appointment. I would also never forgive myself if an urgent matter hides amongst the ring-backs and I would not act on the emergency in time.

Six of the ring-backs are marked 'urine sample'. Those are not urgent and can wait till the end of morning surgery if needed. Another six are marked 'prescription request' and the same applies to those.

One has been marked, 'patient called back'. This suggests the patient was either impatient, deemed the complaint was urgent, or the complaint worsened. I will check that one now to make sure. Twenty-four-year-old Theo phoned complaining of a sore throat and called back to find out when I would phone him back. This one does not appear to be too urgent, and I feel it can wait till later. To help me prioritise the calls appropriately I add the note 'sore throat' to his name on the appointment screen and then direct my attention to the next five ring-backs.

None of these have any message next to them and I open the notes of the first one. Fifty-five-year-old Melissa suffers from a toothache and wants to make certain it is okay to take paracetamol for this. As she is on metformin for diabetes, the dentist has informed her to check with the doctor before using this. The metformin does not cause any problems with the paracetamol, and as there is no other obvious reason in her notes why she couldn't use paracetamol, I send a task to the receptionists to tell her she can. In the same message, I include the maximum dosage she can take safely. However, I fail to understand why the dentist could not have informed her of this instead of directing Melissa to her GP.

* * *

The next ring-back on the screen is from the mum of fourteen-year-old Theo, who suffers from a tummy ache. I send a task to the receptionists to invite him for a sit-and-wait appointment at twenty to eleven. As they already contacted all Dr K's patients for today, they will have more opportunity to act on my tasks now. Sending a task instead of phoning the patient myself, will save me a little time and I can now move on to the next item on my list.

* * *

Thirty-one-year-old Julie believes she has a urine infection and requests antibiotics for this. In response to this ring-back, I send a task to the receptionists to ask Julie to hand a urine sample in so we can check this for her and then act on it appropriately. Another one ticked off on the list for now. At least, until the urine sample lands on my ring-back list.

* * *

As I prepare to move on to the next ring-back, an instant message pops up, "Can you have a look at a patient in my room, please?" The nurse requires my opinion. After I return the message to tell her I'll be with her soon, I check the next ring-back on my list first.

This ring-back is from seventy-two-year-old Barbara, who has an itchy and sore rash she would like checking. This sounds like it could be shingles and I send a task to the receptionists to invite Barbara for a ten past eleven appointment, and to please ask her to wait in a side room in case it is shingles. It is better to avoid contact with other patients in case it is contagious.

* * *

Next, I open the notes for the next ring-back and another instant message pops up, "Urgent prescription in the electronic prescriptions in-box. Can you please sign this?"

When I go to the electronic prescription screen, I find

eighty-three prescriptions waiting and sign them all, then return to the notes of the ring-back. It is already twenty-five past ten and I should definitely hurry a little. I shouldn't keep the patients waiting too long.

Forty-six-year-old Ben wants a sick note as he has suffered from backache since this morning. I send a task to the receptionists to inform Ben he can self-certify if required, but that at this moment a sick note from the doctor is unnecessary. Advice to see us if his symptoms do not improve or if they worsen accompanies my message. And, I also include the advice to seek urgent medical attention if he notices weakness of his legs, numbness down below or if he cannot control his bladder or bowels.

* * *

When I plan to call in the first extra patient, I remember the nurse asked me to see a patient in her room. After logging off from the clinical system, I walk to reception to drop off a few prescriptions I have signed. Next, I join Ruth in her room.

"Thank you for coming. This is twenty-two-year-old Linda, and she has suffered from earache for three days. Can you check if the drum is perforated?"

After checking Linda's ear and making sure the drum is intact, I reassure Linda and Ruth, then return to my room with a bathroom break on the way. My bladder is bursting.

CHAPTER 22

Thursday, 10:35 am

After the quick bathroom break, I return to my room and see the extra patients resulting from the ring-backs. By now it is twenty-five to eleven already and I'm beating myself up over the twenty-five minutes I'm running behind. Although I'm coping with a double workload, it still feels like I'm not doing well enough. Oh, well, beating myself up over this does not help me work any faster or better.

First is thirty-two-year-old Adam, who injured his lower back yesterday while lifting some heavy planters. His wife asked him to move the planters to help her rearrange the garden. Adam did not sustain a fall or any other injuries, but simply pulled his back and now the back hurts on the right-hand side of the lower back.

When I examine Adam, his back is obviously stiff, but there is no evidence he has done anything more than pull his back, a muscle strain. After advising Adam to do exercises known to help with this problem and to use pain relief if he needs this, I talk to him about proper lifting techniques. Always bend your knees, keep your back straight, lift and take the load to where it needs to be. When putting it down, again bend the knees, and keep the back straight. When something is next to you, first turn to face it and then do as described earlier.

Adam is happy with the advice and promises to return if his symptoms don't improve or if they worsen.

* * *

The next patient is seventy-six-year-old Edward, the gentleman with the chesty cough and green phlegm.

"Well, doctor, it started like a normal cold, really. However, over the last week, it seems to have turned and now I'm bringing up this horrible thick and green phlegm. Coming up and down the stairs is a struggle and I sound like an old locomotive when I get upstairs. Can you get me something to clear this?"

I ask Edward a few more questions to get as full a history of his problem as possible. He admits to having smoked twenty cigarettes a day for fifty years, "But I stopped two years ago and haven't touched one since." After complimenting Edward on this achievement, he tells me this is the third time this year already his chest is playing up. The breathlessness is worse at the moment, but Edward has noticed some breathlessness occasionally over the last year.

When I examine his chest, there are crackles on the right side and wheezes on both sides. His oxygen levels are good at 98% and I am satisfied he suffers from a chest infection and requires antibiotics. However, the fact he has been a smoker for fifty years and he has suffered from occasional breathlessness make me wonder if there is more behind his complaint than a simple chest infection. I therefore also give him a form to get a chest X-ray done and arrange for a spirometry (a breathing test) to be done. COPD and lung cancer need to be excluded. Edward's story is highly suspicious of possible chronic bronchitis and the smoking may have caused even more harm than that. After asking him to return for the results of the tests and also if he would not improve or would worsen, Edward leaves.

* * *

Next is twenty-seven-year-old Stephen, with his possibly infected ingrowing toenail. "This toe is hurting like hell, doctor. I need you to do something about it for me."

When I examine the offending toenail, it is ingrowing slightly but there is no redness, swelling or discharge to signify an infection. As I start to explain, a message pops up from Ruth, "Can you come and look at this patient for me, please?" A quick message back to Ruth to tell her I'll be with her shortly, and I continue to explain to Stephen that the toe is not infected and should improve with proper nail care. In other words, don't cut your nails this short again, Stephen.

* * *

Once Stephen has left, I join Ruth in her room to look at sixty-seven-year-old Gladys' leg. Ruth suspects cellulitis (an infection of the skin) and wants my opinion. The left lower leg has an angry red colour, it feels hot to the touch and is swollen. Gladys has a slight temperature of 38.2 and there are no signs this is a blood clot rather than cellulitis. After issuing Gladys with a prescription for antibiotics, which is a rather tricky task as she is on medication which is affected by many types of antibiotics, we advise her to contact us again if no improvement occurs over the next few days, or if it gets worse. In that case, the treatment may need to be changed to antibiotic injections instead of tablet form.

* * *

When I return to my room afterwards, a ring–back marked 'urgent' is waiting for me. Before doing anything else, I open the notes to check the details. "Paramedic with patient. Requesting urgent visit. Please ring ASAP," it reads.

The daughter of eighty–seven–year–old George has phoned an ambulance as he was struggling to breathe and she suspected he needed admission to the hospital. George suffers from severe COPD (chronic bronchitis) and is bringing up thick green phlegm. Even simple activities like putting his clothes on, have George gasping for air. After the paramedic has given me this background information, he then continues to tell me about his oxygen levels, which are only eighty–two at the moment.

Why are they even asking for a visit? George needs to be in the hospital, not to wait for me to do a visit at lunchtime and then admit him to hospital.

"George does not want to be admitted, doctor, and we can't transport him against his wishes. We would, therefore, ask you to come out now to see George as an emergency."

Sorry? Come again. They want me to leave a busy surgery with patients waiting to see me? Only so they are covered if they leave as George does not want to go to hospital? "Sorry, I'm afraid I'm a little overstretched at the moment and will not be able to visit George until later today. But really, he needs to be in hospital with the symptoms and signs you just mentioned."

The paramedic sighs and asks if I can speak to George in that case.

"How are you feeling George?"

"Like a wrung out towel to be honest. But I don't want to go to hospital and be told I'm a time waster." George needs to take a breath every other word, he is really struggling.

"George, it does not sound like you are a time waster. You sound like you need to be in hospital and I would strongly advise you to go with the ambulance which has come for you."

George sounds dejected, "Okay, if you think I need to go to hospital, I will." He still needs to stop every other word to catch his breath.

Pleased to have convinced George to do what is best for him, I continue to the next item on the list.

* * *

At ten past eleven, twelve-year-old Kimberley and her mum come in. The appointment was planned for half-past ten and with all the interruptions and the workload, I'm now running forty minutes behind schedule. I hate days like this, where I struggle to remain in control and don't run on time. Where whatever I do simply is not enough to achieve that, "Come in, have a seat. I'm sorry to keep you waiting, it's one of those days."

Kimberley started her periods a year ago and mum describes them as heavy and requests something to help Kimberley with this.

When I ask Kimberley how often she needs to change her pads, she shrugs her shoulders. It's not that bad, is it? "Twice during the day and once at nighttime," she then adds.

Another case of unrealistic expectations. Patiently, I explain that Kimberley's periods are not excessively heavy and that they require no medication for them. Even when I tell mum most women need to change more often than that, she seems unconvinced. Now I am curious. What are mum's periods like?

"I dunno really. They used to be as heavy as Kimberley's, I guess, but since I had Kimberley, my periods stopped altogether."

That explains a lot. If mum is measuring Kimberley's periods against her non-existent ones, then yes Kimberley would be heavy.

Kimberley waves the back of her hand at mum, "I told you so, but you wouldn't listen."

Still arguing, they leave the room.

* * *

At twenty past eleven, fourteen-year-old Theo attends with his mum. Although Dr K's eighth patient for twenty past eleven has also arrived, I see Theo first. He has been waiting the longest after all.

"Yesterday morning Theo started vomiting. This has settled, but now he has diarrhoea," mum turns her eyes on me expectantly like she wants to say 'now do something about that.'

When I ask a few questions, it turns out that Theo has a cramping tummy ache. Mum feels this is abnormal and should be sorted. I suspect it is because of the gastroenteritis he most likely suffers from, in other words, a tummy bug.

During the examination, I find no abnormalities. Theo's stomach is soft and does not hurt when I touch it. There are no lumps or bumps that shouldn't be there and I conclude he indeed has a tummy bug.

After explaining this to mum and Theo and advising to drink plenty of fluids and eat if he wishes and as long as it doesn't upset his stomach, they leave, promising to return if symptoms worsen or don't improve.

* * *

Next is seventy-two-year-old Barbara with her itchy and sore rash. She has been waiting in the side room as requested and I now have a chance to ask her more about the rash and check it. Hopefully, I will be able to see Dr K's patient after her as I should have a little gap before the next extra patient is due to arrive.

"Well, I had this itch on the left side of my stomach and back for about two days. When I itched it, it hurt, really hot and like burning needles. And yesterday this rash appeared," Barbara lifts her jumper and shows me a blistery rash around her waist on the left, the background is red and this indeed looks like shingles. "Look."

The second one this week. Although you can't catch shingles from shingles, there were still two cases this week on my watch. Again I explain what shingles is, and that treatment is only aimed at avoiding persisting pain after the rash disappears. Barbara leaves with a prescription of acyclovir, an antiviral medication and she will get in touch if she needs anything for the pain.

* * *

By now it is half-past eleven and thirty-eight-year-old David is not impressed I kept him waiting or to be seeing me instead of Dr K. Again I apologise for the delay and explain Dr K is currently off sick.

David attends the surgery for a review of his depression and needs another sick note. For the sake of the sick note, he is willing to put up with me, "Don't expect me to go over the entire story again. Dr K already knows all about it and I don't want to tell you again."

Instead, I ask David if his symptoms have improved, stayed the same or worsened and he tells me there is not much improvement. He denies suicidal thoughts and I give him a note for another four weeks. This also appears to be the duration of the previous notes.

* * *

Now David has left, I prepare to take a quick look through the waiting ring-backs. A message from the nurse pops up on my screen, "Can you come to my room again, please?" The ring-backs will have to wait.

Forty-five-year-old Mandy came to see the nurse regarding a painful tongue, but Ruth could not find much to account for the symptoms.

When I examine Mandy's tongue there is a very slight white coating on it, suggestive of thrush and I issue a prescription for nystatin suspension to cure this, telling Mandy to return if her symptoms don't improve.

* * *

When I return to my room, it is twenty to twelve. Time to check the ring-backs.

The fourteenth ring-back is from twenty-seven-year-old Amy, who is seven weeks pregnant and has started bleeding. The bleeding is accompanied by some cramps in her lower stomach, which Amy describes as being a bit like period pains. At the moment there is only a little blood, less than during a period but Amy is understandably anxious, "Am I having a miscarriage? Should I go to A&E?"

Unfortunately, there is nothing that can stop a miscarriage if Amy is having one. The blood loss combined with the period-like pain makes this a distinct possibility, but nothing the medical profession does will stop it from happening.

"At the moment, I can't tell you if you are having a miscarriage or not. If, and that is only if, you are having a miscarriage, there is nothing we can do to stop that from happening," I take a breath, "As you are only bleeding a little, this is not a medical emergency and therefore you don't need go to casualty at the moment. All you can do for now, is to take it easy and hope for the best. In the meantime, I will contact the hospital and try to get you an appointment in the Early Pregnancy Assessment Unit. This will probably be tomorrow at the earliest, but it can be a few days before they have an appointment available. They will hopefully be in a better position to tell you what is happening. So, I will phone them as soon as we put down the phone and I'll call you back with the outcome. Is that okay?"

Amy agrees, and I put down the phone. Next, I phone the hospital and ask switchboard to put me through to the Early Pregnancy Assessment Unit (EPAU). I explain the situation and the next available appointment is at ten tomorrow morning. Amy is lucky, the patient I referred two weeks ago had to wait three days for her appointment. Although it makes no difference to the outcome, it does make a difference to the mental state of the patient.

"Amy?" She confirms it's her. "I have spoken to the hospital and they have an appointment available for you tomorrow morning at ten. For this appointment you will need to bring an urine sample and the letter I will write for you. If you can come by the surgery to pick the letter up later today, that would be great. Good luck, I hope everything will be alright for you."

After we hang up, I write a quick letter and put it to the side to take to reception later. Hopefully, this is just a false alarm.

* * *

The next ring-back is from the grandma of two-year-old Amy, who is complaining of a sore throat, has a temperature and a snotty nose. Grandma is asking for Amy to be checked over. A task to offer a twenty past twelve sit and wait appointment makes its way to the receptionists and I turn my attention to the next problem.

* * *

Next is a ring-back is for a prescription request for a resident of a nursing home. The patient suffers from dry skin and often uses E45; they have requested another prescription for this cream. After issuing the prescription, I still wonder why the receptionist did not send the request as a task instead, I send a task to inform them the prescription is ready. Certainly, a request for a cream which is also available over the counter is not an urgent problem.

* * *

By now it is twelve and my stomach is rumbling. Still, work comes first. This ring- back is also a prescription request, a nursing home is requesting paracetamol for a patient with pain in his hip. At the moment he is not taking anything for pain yet and paracetamol is the appropriate medication to try first. After issuing a prescription, I send a task to the receptionists to inform the home and advise to review if the pain relief is insufficient.

* * *

On to the next prescription request. Eighty-five-year-old Vernon suffers with COPD and has a self-management plan. Yesterday he started the antibiotics he has on standby for chest infections and he is now requesting another course of antibiotics to keep on standby for the next chest infection. Vernon's current course was issued nine months ago, so there are no signs of over usage. I issue the prescription and send a task to inform the patient and to advise him to contact us if his symptoms don't improve or worsen. If any appointments are available for our minor illness nurse or one of the doctors, I would prefer if Ruth or a doctor could see Vernon during his current infection too.

* * *

Now I move on to the next ring-back marked as

prescription request. Am I starting to regain some control? It is too early to know for certain. Still, I have returned several ring-backs and some weight is lifting from my chest and the invisible hand lets go of my throat.

Twenty-seven-year-old Tom is requesting an urgent prescription for his blue inhaler, his Ventolin. Tom is a known asthmatic and when I check the notes, he is overdue his annual asthma review. However, I can't withhold the inhaler until he attends a review appointment and issue the prescription, sending a task to the receptionists to inform him of this and to book him an appointment for a review with the nurse. Hopefully, he will attend. Too often patients will be 'too busy' to attend and unwittingly take unnecessary risks with their life. Asthma can potentially kill if not taken serious. Tom also appears to have rather frequent prescriptions for ventolin which suggests uncontrolled asthma. This is an indication a review is paramount in Tom's case.

* * *

The next ring-back brings a prescription request from the district nurse. She has visited eighty-three-year-old Peter, who is in the end stages of terminal bowel cancer. At the moment he receives his pain relief and anti-sickness medication via a syringe driver, a continuous infusion directly under his skin. One of my colleagues saw Peter within the last week and Trish requests another prescription for his medication and another syringe driver instruction for him. These instructions need to be updated every five days.

After issuing, printing and signing the prescriptions, I fill in the instructions and print those off too. For now, I put them to the side to take to reception later and send a task to the receptionists to inform them they are ready.

* * *

There is another prescription request from the district nurse. Trish believes an elderly lady has cellulitis, and she has requested a prescription for antibiotics. Although Trish is generally spot on with her diagnoses, I ring her to double-check her findings. She informs me of the redness, heat and swelling of the patient's right lower leg, the leg does not feel tight and hard and she is convinced there is no sign of a blood clot. From her description it indeed appears to only be cellulitis and I issue the requested prescription, advising to seek medical attention if the symptoms do not improve or worsen. Trish promises to visit the patient again in two days and the patient's relatives will collect the prescription from reception later and contact us if any problems occur in the interim.

* * *

When I check the appointment screen, no further patients arrived during my time signing the prescription requests. The next one should be the twenty-past-twelve sit-and-wait patient. Reassured I have time to, I scan through the remaining ring-backs. At the moment, only urine sample results are waiting for my input.

The first urine sample is from twenty-four-year-old Lacey, who believes she has a urine infection, she has no allergies and is not known to be pregnant. The urine sample is clear, and I send a task to inform the patient of this. She does not suffer from a urine infection at the moment. However, if her symptoms persist, she should book an appointment with a doctor or our minor illness nurse.

* * *

Twenty-three minutes past twelve and the extra patient has still not arrived yet. Instead, I move on to the next urine sample.

This one is again for a suspected urine infection. The

sample of thirty-seven-year-old Angela is clear and again a task makes its way to the receptionists to inform her of this, including the safety-netting.

Safety-netting is how we try to put a safety net under any advice we give to ensure a patient seeks further help if the symptoms don't improve. What seems common sense to most is not to everyone. Often, even when symptoms worsen, patients continue to cling to the reassurance given at the time they attended the surgery. Instead, they should seek further medical attention when symptoms don't improve, and if they worsen or change. Doctors don't have a crystal ball and cannot predict any changes which may take place after the patient leaves the consulting room.

* * *

The next urine sample is from eighty-three-year-old Georgina and shows signs of infection. Georgina has no medication which would interact with antibiotics, no allergies, and her last urine infection was many years ago when she was in her fifties. I issue a prescription for nitrofurantoin, the first line antibiotic for a suspected urine infection in the elderly. Next, I send a task to inform her of this and to advise her to contact us if her symptoms don't improve or worsen.

* * *

There are only a few more urine samples left to assess. The extra patient has arrived in the meantime, but I will first clear the few urine samples left.

This one is from seventy-eight-year-old Bill, who has frequent urine infections and is under the care of the urologist (waterworks specialist) for this. The sample is not conclusive. Only a trace of leucocytes (white blood cells which deal with infection) and no other abnormalities are present in the sample. When I look through the details surrounding the sample, I find Bill has only observed a pungent smell before he brought a urine sample to the surgery but suffers no other symptoms suggestive of a urine infection.

In view of his frequent infections, I prefer to wait for the culture results to return from the hospital first, and to have confirmation this is an infection. I send a task to inform Bill of this and to advise him to contact us if his symptoms worsen. In that case, we would need to treat him blind (without the benefit of the culture and sensitivities report) after all. To know what we are dealing with first, and which antibiotic is likely to get rid of it, is preferable though.

* * *

At nearly half-past twelve it is time for the fifth urine sample. This one is from thirty-two-year-old pregnant Lydia. The sample suggests a urine infection and I prepare a prescription for amoxicillin as this is safe in pregnancy. With the advice to contact us if the symptoms worsen or don't improve included in the task, I move on to the next problem on my list.

* * *

Twenty-nine minutes to one. I'm feeling a little restless and my right leg moves up and down as I urge myself to go faster. After this urine sample I will still need to see the last extra patient of the morning and I should have been in our weekly meeting already. This urine sample is from fifty-six-year-old Daryl, who has had no known previous urine infection. This sample is, however, suggestive of infection and as he has no known allergies, I issue a prescription, send a task and advise him to book an appointment with a doctor if he has any further urine infections, does not improve or worsens. If any man has more than one urine infection, this needs to be investigated further.

* * *

Another urine sample. Thirty-one-year-old Julie has

brought in the sample as requested, and this is clear. Another task finds its way to the receptionists to inform Julie of this. Her suspicion of a urine infection is proven incorrect.

* * *

Finally! At twenty-five to one, I call in two-year-old Amy and her grandma. Amy seems a little off colour, pale and clingy.

"Amy has been off it for the last two days, doctor. My daughter and I are really worried about her. Today, Amy has not eaten anything, and she is drinking very little."

When I check her throat, her tonsils are up and have white spots all over them. The glands in Amy's neck are up and although she has had Calpol (paracetamol) only half an hour ago, her temperature is up at 38.3. With a diagnosis of tonsillitis made, I prepare a prescription for antibiotics and hand this to grandma.

"Please, give this to Amy three times a day."

I turn to Amy, "Do you like ice cream?"

Her eyes sparkle at the word ice cream and she nods her head.

"Ice cream may help to soothe Amy's throat, anything cold can so it may be worth a try."

Grandma nods and with the advice to seek medical

attention if Amy doesn't improve or if she worsens, grandma thanks me, puts Amy on her hip and leaves the room.

* * *

A quarter to one and I am desperate to get to the meeting. I hate being late, and knowing people are waiting for me. An earlier ring-back has been put back on the list again. Forty-six-year-old Ben with his backache wants to have an appointment today. Now it is not about his sick note, but the pain is such that he wishes to have an appointment today. Ben has no history of injuries. With the meeting eating up my lunchtime and the fact that Baby Clinic is due to start at two, there is no chance to see Ben before surgery starts this afternoon. Instead, I offer a ten past five sit and wait appointment for after the normal surgery this afternoon. I really need to hurry now.

* * *

Now it is finally time to get to the meeting. On the way, I drop off the prescriptions and forms at reception, then go to the bathroom and afterwards pick up my lunch to join my colleague and the practice manager. Will Dr K have made it or is he still not well enough to be at work? If he isn't well enough yet, I must cope with being duty doctor and running Baby Clinic at the same time.

CHAPTER 23

Thursday, 12:48 pm

When I arrive in the meeting room, Angela, Linda and Dr K are already waiting. Dr P is on holiday this week and won't attend the weekly meeting.

"Sorry to keep you waiting, it's been a little hectic this morning."

Angela looks at me over the rim of her glasses, "Yes, you have had a busy morning, haven't you?"

Dr K glances over, "Sorry, I had an awful migraine this morning and simply couldn't make it."

I'm glad Dr K is here now, otherwise I would need to cope with both Baby Clinic and duty this afternoon. "Feeling better?"

Dr K nods, "Yes, thank you, much better after sleeping a few hours this morning."

"Well, if you need any help, you know where to find me." Hopefully, Dr K will manage without my help.

Angela clears her throat, "We should get started, there is a lot on the agenda today and Baby Clinic starts again at two."

* * *

Angela opens the meeting by making sure we are happy with the notes from the last meeting and follows on with the outstanding issues from previous meetings.

"Okay, so the soap dispensers we ordered to replace the malfunctioning ones, have arrived. Jeremy will fit them in the toilets next week."

Jeremy is our handyman, who comes to sort out any little bits that need fixing on a weekly basis. He also performs the weekly fire alarm test and checks things like the hot water storage and a few other things. Jeremy is basically our maintenance guy.

"Next item is the fax machine. After you all agreed last week, this has been ordered and it should arrive next week." The current fax machine is rather temperamental and occasionally eats the paper instead of printing it. Although it is something that is still manageable, it is annoying and we are waiting for the day to come when it completely gives up the will to live.

"Last but not least, I ordered the keys to the building and they will soon arrive so Dr P can also get a set." Angela leafs through her notes, "Yes, I think that covers all the outstanding items."

* * *

A glance at my watch tells me it is almost one already.
"Time to move on to staff issues. Patricia will retire in
three months and we need to decide whether to recruit
another member of staff or do a reshuffle. I looked at
how things are at the moment and I would suggest we
recruit someone to cover Patricia's duties and add
some hours on top as a floater in case someone is on
holiday."

Dr K's head comes up.

"Now, before you say anything, I know this will be a
larger expense, but it will help the running of the
practice in the longer term. It will also give us the
opportunity to consider taking on extra services
offered by the CCG and therefore bring more money
into the practice." Angela checks her papers again, "In
the near future, the CCG is planning to offer an
expansion of services that are currently provided by
hospital to take place in primary care instead.
Although we are overstretched already, the extra
money this will bring, would help to pay for the extra
hours of receptionist's time. You don't need to decide
today, but think about it."

Both Dr K and I mumble something about how

overstretched we are already and that no amount of money weighs up to the extra work and pressure this will bring.

"I'm sorry, but we may not have a choice in the matter. If the services are no longer provided by secondary care, then we will need to offer them."

Oh joy, the pleasures of being self-employed and being the boss. Still being ruled by the powers that be.

Angela moves on to the next item on the agenda, Elaine will have worked at the practice for twenty years next month and she wonders how we would acknowledge this achievement. We toss ideas about. Perhaps we could get her a present, something like a watch or bracelet or something like that, or maybe a voucher so she can pick her own gift. Another option could be to offer an extra week of holiday on top of her normal holiday entitlement. Although we come up with several ideas, a decision can't be made today. Dr P should have a say in the staff issues too.

Now that we have discussed the staffing issues, Angela moves on to the next item, "The fridge in the kitchen is not working properly, the seal no longer works and milk has gone off overnight. Can we replace the fridge please?"

That sounds like a good idea, most people working at the practice use milk in their tea or coffee, I am the odd one out. We ask Angela to get some quotes and we can then decide based on those quotes.

* * *

Angela moves on to the finances, "Over the last few weeks, I have looked at places where we could make some savings. Insurance, electricity, gas and telephone charges may be areas where we can make savings. Can I look into this further and make changes if these are appropriate?"

Dr K and I agree with Angela looking into these possible savings, we would like to have the last say in the matter. Insurance can be a difficult area as there are a few things we need to consider. For instance, our lease agreement insists on the insurance being approved by the owner of the building.

"There are also a few contract changes you need to be aware of. The smoking cessation provision will be removed from individual practices in three months and a regional body will take this service over. Although in principle we could continue to provide the service, they will no longer pay for this service. This would mean we would pay our smoking cessation adviser out of our own pocket with no reimbursement.

We agree it would be best to stop providing the service in that case, but need to have Dr P's agreement on this too. I don't foresee any problems with that.

As I face Angela, I realise we need to make sure our staff member involved should be kept up to date on the developments, "Can you please make sure our smoking cessation adviser is aware of the changes about to take place? She needs to know that part of her job will soon end."

Next, Angela brings up a new service the CCG is expecting from practices. All practices have to sign up to this service and we need to set out our plans of how we believe we can provide that service. The aim of the service is to ensure that vulnerable patients get the attention they need and that we avoid unnecessary admissions to hospital.

To do this, we first need to set up a register of patients who we consider being vulnerable and at risk of emergency admissions. A tool is available to find some of these patients based on admission details kept by the hospital. Any patients with frequent admissions are potential candidates for the register.

The requirement for this register is that it should be at least two percent of the entire practice population, which in our case means there should be about one hundred and fifty patients on that list. Each and every patient on the list should be seen by a GP to set up a personal care plan. As part of this personal care plan, we need to discuss several things with the patient and potentially their family. Several of those things are rather difficult to discuss. First, we need to consider why the patient is at risk of admission. What illnesses does the patient suffer from and what can we do to avoid the illnesses becoming that unstable that an admission is needed? Where would a patient prefer to be treated? At home? In a nursing home? In hospital? The more tricky discussions revolve around end-of-life care and dying. What treatment does the patient want to receive and what does the patient consider too much? Where does the patient prefer to die? Does the patient want to be resuscitated?

To set up a care plan will take at least twenty minutes for each and every individual patient on the list and we decide we will use the last appointments on a morning or afternoon for this reason. I suspect in most cases the discussion will take over half an hour. This is all on top of our already heavy workload.

Not all the patients will be able to attend the surgery and we may need to do several home visits for these reviews instead. Many of our vulnerable patients will be housebound. This puts another twenty minutes on top of the time already required.

The next part of the service is the need to review these patients whenever they needed to attend A&E or were admitted to hospital as an emergency. Changes to the care plan may need to take place at that point and a new care plan printed and handed to the patient. If no admissions or A&E attendances have taken place, the patient still needs a review every three to six months, anyway.

The last part of the service is the need to report to the CCG every three months to show we have done our job, and the service has made an impact, a reduction in the A&E attendance and emergency admission rate has taken place. Whether this will lead to an actual reduction in admissions and attendances is doubtful, but we are obliged to take part. This is considered good practice and overstretched or not, we will need to make provisions for this service to take place.

Our discussions centre around how to identify the vulnerable patients, how long the appointments should be, where we should place those appointments, how to spread the work over the three doctors in the practice and whether we can involve the practice nurses in this too. All care plans should be completed within three months, but half within the first month. What do they think we are? Miracle workers? My watch tells me we need to rush, baby clinic should start any minute now and I get rather edgy. At several points I drop the fact I need to get back to surgery, but still they need me to stay. It is nearly two and we still have to discuss one more thing.

* * *

The remainder of the meeting we spend discussing significant events. Anything that had gone wrong, nearly went wrong or could have gone wrong but was put right before it did.

I keep a close eye on my watch, time is ticking on and it is already nearly two. Only a few minutes left until I need to get back to seeing patients.

The first problem we discuss is a lady who visited the surgery uninvited. After she sat in the waiting area for a few minutes, she got up, made for the door between the waiting area and the hall leading to the consulting rooms and simply sauntered through it. Trish was at reception at the time and got up to follow her. The lady moved fast and already moved through another door leading up the stairs, where another member of staff unlocked the door to the upstairs offices. She simply followed the staff member in and marched to an office door to open this. By then, Trish caught up with her, "Excuse me, can I help you?"

The woman informed her she came to an appointment with a friend and was now looking for her. When Trish queried who the patient was, and the woman gave a name, not fitting any patients due to be seen that day, or even any known patient, she pushed Trish aside and ran through another door downstairs and out of the building.

In recent weeks, e-mails from other practices about someone with this woman's description had circulated and items had gone missing from handbags of members of staff.

We discussed what went well. The fact Trish confronted the woman about what she was doing in a restricted area of the building and that she left was positive. But the woman had gained access to the restricted area of the building and walked past the receptionist, and that should not have happened.

Next, we discussed what we should do to try to avoid this happening in the future. We only came up with the plan to investigate how much it would cost to place a lock on the connecting door between the waiting area and the consulting rooms. If this was something affordable and would not cause too much disruption to the receptionist's other tasks, we should consider this. For now, we agreed to be vigilant and even more careful not to leave any handbags where others might gain access to them. Fortunately, I already have my bags behind lock and key, anyway.

When Angela wants to discuss another case, I become

more insistent, "Sorry, I really need to get downstairs. It's ten past two and Baby Clinic has started already. I have to go." I get up and leave, using the bathroom before starting Baby Clinic.

* * *

When I return to my room, I put away the lunchbox, pour tea into my cup and log onto the computer again. Another four ring-backs arrived during my absence, but none are marked urgent. They will need to wait until after surgery or until I have a break between patients. Even though I know it was right to return downstairs for baby clinic, I still feel guilty for having left the meeting before it finished.

CHAPTER 24

Thursday, 2:18 pm

I love Baby Clinic, or Well-Baby Clinic as we officially call it. During Baby Clinic we see babies for their eight-week check or their heart checks at the age of one. The little cuddles and playing with the little ones always make me happier and also make me broody. Yes, I know, I already have four children.

The first one on the screen is eight-week-old Joshua, who has come with his parents. His beaming mum and dad enter the room with Joshua in his car seat.

"Congratulations. How is everything going? Do you enjoy being parents?"

Their smiles become even wider and their eyes shine as Joshua's parents confirm they love being parents.

So far, they have encountered no problems. Joshua feeds well, he is breast-fed, and he smiles and follows movements.

Now it is time for Joshua's check. Mum carries him to the couch, closely followed by Dad, and undresses Joshua, leaving his nappy on at my request. In the meantime I wash my hands and grab a stethoscope and ophthalmoscope (a tool to look into eyes with). For the checks, I start at the top and work my way down the body. His soft spot feels normal, his eyes are open, and he follows where mum goes. When I glance in Joshua's eyes, the light reflex is normal. Joshua's mouth seems normal, his neck and shoulders too. He has two arms with hands and the expected number of fingers. The heart sounds normal and the lungs too. Joshua's tummy shows no abnormalities and there is no evidence of a hernia. Both hips are stable. When I check his private area, all is in order there as well and his testicles have descended (a real feat considering my hands are usually freezing cold). Joshua's legs, feet and toes are fine and all reflexes are normal. Now I turn Joshua over and a check of his back is also unremarkable. He has a 'stork bite' though, a little birthmark at the nape of his neck.

 The last thing I check is mostly for the benefit of the parents. When babies are this young, they often still have an old 'walking-reflex'. I lift Joshua and let the top of one of his feet touch the couch. Yes, as expected Joshua lifts the foot and places it on the couch, the next foot follows and he takes a few steps. His parents absolutely beam at their brilliant son.

Now that Joshua has passed his first check with us

with flying colours, mum dresses him again while I enter all the details of the examination on the records.

* * *

Next is eight-week-old Millie who attends with mum and grandma. Mum Olivia is only seventeen herself and lives with her parents. Dad is no longer on the scene; as soon as he found out he would become a dad, he did a runner.

"Congratulations. Did everything go okay with the birth?"

Olivia nods.

"Are you enjoying being a mum?"

Olivia nods again.

When I ask if they have any concerns, grandma points to a rash on Millie's face, "Millie has rather dry skin and we wonder what it is and should be done about it."

After promising to look at it while I examine Millie, Olivia tells me Millie takes her bottles well and there are no further problems or worries.

Just like with Joshua, I check Millie from top to bottom and other than the rash, a mild form of eczema, I find no abnormalities during the examination. I advise them to use a mild moisturiser and prepare a prescription for that, then it is time for Millie to see the nurse for her vaccinations.

* * *

The third baby today is eight-week-old Billy, who comes with both parents. Billy is also breastfed and appears to do everything expected from him. His parents have no concerns.

The same routine follows for Billy's examination and soon I declare him fit too. Billy will see the nurse for his jabs when he leaves my room.

* * *

By now it is ten to three, and I have nearly caught up. The appointment for eight-week-old Max was due at a quarter to three. Both parents accompany Max to the appointment, he is breast-fed and they have so far not noticed any problems. The first check in hospital after the birth was entirely normal.

When I examine Max, he appears to be completely healthy. A listen to his heart reveals a murmur, but it sounds like this is an innocent murmur. After reassuring the parents the murmur likely is innocent, I explain I will refer Max for a paediatric opinion as I don't like taking chances. I don't expect any problems, though.

His parents agree to the referral and leave to book the appointment at reception.

* * *

Before moving on to the next patient, I first write a letter to the paediatrician for Max. In this letter I mention all the details given by the parents, details about the murmur and my suspicion this is an innocent murmur. When the letter is ready, I send a task to the secretary to send the letter electronically as soon as the appointment has been booked.

Now it is time to move on to the next patient.

* * *

The fifth baby was due at three and toddles in at eight past three. One-year-old Bobby dawdles into the consultation room supported by Mum. Mum holds onto both of Bobby's hands as he places one foot in front of the other. That is one question answered, Bobby is definitely starting to walk.

At the age of one, we check the basic development. Things like attempting to walk and talk. Bobby speaks a few small words, Mum, Dad, Rover (the dog), and Mum has no concerns about him or his development.

The other things we do at this age, is to listen to the heart sounds and feel the pulses in the groin. In Bobby's case, everything is fine and his next stop is the nurse for his vaccinations.

* * *

The last baby to be seen in Baby Clinic today, is one-year-old Macey. Grandma has come with her today as mum has to work and also doesn't enjoy being present for Macey's vaccinations. There are no concerns about Macey's development or health, she walks, speaks some words and is quite active. When I listen to her heart and feel the pulses in her groin, they also appear normal. Another healthy baby.

* * *

By now it is twenty-five past three and normal surgery is due to start in a few minutes. From half-past three until five, I have a normal booked surgery and I already know there will be one extra patient and a few ring-backs for me to complete afterwards. For now, it is time to take a quick bathroom break before I get started with surgery. The babies put a smile on my face again and lifted my spirit. I feel ready to cope with the rest of the afternoon again.

CHAPTER 25

Thursday, 3:30 pm

At half-past three, following Baby Clinic, I have another surgery until five. Whenever I'm the doctor in charge of Baby Clinic, the plan is to finish early at five instead of half-past five with the afternoon surgery. Today I already know life won't be that easy. After all, I was on call in the morning and a few ring-backs still remain and at least one extra patient is left over from my on call.

My first patient for the afternoon surgery is sixty-seven-year-old Philip, who has noticed a lump on his left wrist for the last four months. Over this time, the lump has slowly increased in size, Philip tells me, but it has not caused him any problems. He is only concerned about its presence and what this would mean, the ever-present question in the back of his mind, "could this be cancer?"

"And this lump is not causing you any problems?"

Philip nods, "That's right doctor. No pain or discomfort. I just want to know what it is and how to get rid of the lump."

When I examine the lump it is located directly over the back of his left wrist, exactly over the joints. The lump feels solid, but not hard and from the way it is presenting, it is obvious this is what we call a ganglion. Ganglions are innocent swellings over joints, a little like a cyst. These are part of the joint capsule, only they have kind of prolapsed between the little bones in the wrist.

I face Philip again, "This is what we call a ganglion. Have you heard of those?"

Philip shakes his head and I explain what a ganglion is.

"A lot of years ago, people would pick up one of those large and heavy bibles and hit the lump with it to get rid of them. As you can imagine, we don't do that any longer. Even if we would, the lump would likely return anyway," I take a breath and continue, "Ganglions are absolutely innocent and require no treatment. If, however, the lump would cause you any problems, I could refer you to the orthopaedic surgeons. Removal is possible, but they often return. The ganglions are part of the ageing of the joint."

Philip is happy to find out the lump is not cancer and pleased with the explanation he leaves. He will return if the lump causes him any problems, and that is quite unlikely.

* * *

 The consultation with Philip only took five minutes of my time and this leaves me with a short amount of time to check one of the ring-backs.
 The mother of five-year-old Megan would like her to be examined. Megan returned from nursery with a temperature, a snotty nose and a cough. Although Megan may be absolutely fine with a simple cold, I send a task to the receptionists to invite Megan for a twenty past five sit and wait appointment.

* * *

 As I still have another few minutes left before the next patient is due, I look at the next ring-back. Thirty-four-year-old Melanie has an unplanned pregnancy and would like to be seen today. When a request like that arrives, it usually means the pregnancy is unwanted as well as unplanned and the patient would like to request a termination of pregnancy. The other doctors in the surgery refuse to refer a patient for this, which means all these patients will end up on my list, anyway. For myself, I may not agree with abortions, but I do strongly believe in the patient's right to make that choice for themselves. Obviously, supported by the people around them to ensure it is the right decision for that patient. Bearing this in mind, I send a task to the receptionists to invite her for a sit-and-wait appointment at half-past five.

* * *

The next ring-back is for forty-three-year-old Malcolm, who is complaining of a painful scrotum and wishes to be seen for this. A complaint like that could mean anything. From an infection of his epididymis, to a twisted testicle, to an injury during sports. In view of this, I send a task to the receptionists to invite him for a sit and wait appointment at twenty to six. This is going to be another long day, it seems.

* * *

The last ring-back on the list is for eighty-four-year-old Leslie. Leslie's daughter phoned as she is concerned about her father's memory problems and she would like to speak to a doctor about this today. This ring-back is likely to be difficult and I decide to leave it until after the surgery today. Now, I need to see the next patient on my booked list this afternoon.

* * *

Fifty-six-year-old Janet has come for an annual medication review. Janet takes seven different medications a day and these need to be reviewed annually. The first medication is bendroflumethiazide, a water tablet used for the control of her blood pressure. Janet has no problems tolerating the medication and her blood pressure is well controlled, a sign the medication is doing its job. Her blood results are normal, kidney function tests, liver function tests and sugar level are all within the normal or target levels. Her cholesterol is a little above target at 5.6 and we will need to look at that later.

Next on the list is amlodipine, another blood pressure medication. Janet reports no problems with this one either and we move on to the next medication on the list.

She has been taking lansoprazole for acid reflux for several months and no longer has any symptoms of this. Janet also has lost weight and is now at a healthy weight, she has stopped smoking and avoids spicy food and alcohol. "Do you think I could reduce this medication and maybe even stop taking it?" Janet has a hopeful expression in her eyes.

"That sounds like a good idea. In the first instance we can reduce it to half the dose you are currently taking, and perhaps in a few months' time we can try to stop it completely." We agree on this course of action and I make the necessary changes on her repeat list and issue a prescription for the lower dose medication.

Janet has also been taking HRT for the last six years. The advice is to take this for a maximum of five years and Janet agrees to reduce and stop this. She still has a two-month supply at home and will not request another prescription once this runs out. The HRT is removed from the repeat list.

Four medications reviewed, three more to go. The next one on the list is a painkiller. Janet rarely uses this and the last prescription issued was over a year ago. We agree to remove this one from the list as well and Janet will return if she needs pain relief in the future.

The sixth medication on her list is something for an overactive bladder. It works well for her and Janet tolerates is well.

Last but not least is her cholesterol tablet, simvastatin. "There was something on the news this week about the medication increasing blood sugar levels. Should I be concerned about that?"

Once again, I explain how the risks of a small increase in sugar levels are far outweighed by the risks of Janet having a heart attack or stroke if she did not take the medication.

"I guess I should continue to take the tablets then."

This brings us to the next point on the list. Janet's cholesterol was above target. "Actually, we need to have a little discussion about your cholesterol. When we last checked your cholesterol level, it was 5.6 which is above the recommended level of five for someone with your risk factors. I would, therefore, recommend we increase your simvastatin to forty milligrams daily instead of twenty."

Janet and I discuss briefly if there are any other actions she can take other than increasing the dose of the tablets, but she is already very strict with her diet and no further improvements appear to be possible. She agrees to the increase in the dose and after advising her to repeat the cholesterol levels and liver function test six weeks after the increase, the change is made to her repeat list and the medication issued.

* * *

Henry is a forty-four-year-old, who comes to see me today with a painful left elbow, "My elbow has been hurting for the last two months. I expected it would get better, but it still is no better. In fact, it is getting worse. So, I have come to you to tell me what's wrong."

Henry denies any injuries. He is a manual labourer,

and the problem is causing him some trouble at work, "The gaffer told me to go to my doctor or face a disciplinary, so here I am."

When I examine his left elbow, there is no swelling, redness, and there are no other distinguishable features. However, when I put pressure on the insertion of the tendons at the elbow, these hurt a lot, "Ah, you have tennis elbow, Henry," and I explain what this means and that the problem can last a few months.

Henry is not impressed, "Surely you can do something about that. I need to work and don't want to get in trouble with the gaffer."

After discussing the matter a while longer, we agree Henry will talk with his manager and if needed we can give him a note for amended duties. Now feeling happier, Henry leaves again.

* * *

This afternoon is turning into a bit of an orthopaedic one. First, the ganglion, then a tennis elbow and now twenty-eight-year-old Lucy has come with problems with her left arm and hand.

"I keep having pins and needles in my left hand all the time. It hurts and sometimes keeps me awake at night."

When I ask Lucy a few more questions, she tells me the symptoms are mainly in her thumb, index finger and middle finger. At night she will have to shake her hand to get the feeling back in it and it aches all the time.

Lucy's symptoms are highly suggestive of carpal tunnel syndrome and when I apply pressure on the palm side of her wrist, her symptoms worsen.

"In carpal tunnel syndrome, the nerve that supplies that part of your hand," I point to the fingers affected, "gets trapped in the carpal tunnel. This is a tunnel formed between the bones of the wrist and a little fibrous band which keeps those together."

After further explanations about which circumstances make it worse, like pregnancy, warmth, obesity, we agree her symptoms are such that she would like treatment for it.

"Before even considering surgery, we have a much simpler option we can try first. This is often quite successful." I excuse myself and go to reception to collect a splint. "Let's try this." Now I fit the splint around Lucy's left wrist and immobilise the wrist. This will often improve the symptoms and allow swelling around the carpal tunnel to recede. "How does that seem? Not too tight?"

Lucy tells me it appears to be fine.

"Now, wear the splint at night and hopefully that should help the symptoms to improve. I would like you to return for a review in about six weeks, but you are free to return earlier if needed."

With that, Lucy leaves the room, already looking happier.

* * *

My next patient is thirty-four-year-old Emily, who has come with her partner. Emily has tried to conceive for the last eighteen months and not been successful. Emily and Tony are now worried something might be wrong with one of them and would like to find out more.

"I take it you are not using any contraception?" The problem earlier this week has shown me not to take anything for granted.

Disbelief shows on their faces as their mouths open and eyes widen, "Of course not, we're not stupid." I explain that it is always best to first make sure of the basics.

Tony and Emily are both healthy individuals, no infections in the area and Tony has not suffered mumps either.

After explaining it sometimes takes longer to get pregnant and the fact they have not managed to so far does not necessarily mean anything is wrong, we agree to get a few initial investigations set up.

"Let's organise some blood tests for you, Emily and also a few swabs to ensure you carry no infections." Ensuring this is essential if we would consider referral for their problem. I turn towards Tony, "And for you, we need to arrange a sperm count."

After filling the required forms and handing them to the couple, I explain what they need to do and advise Emily and Tony to return after the tests have been done for the results. At that time we can also decide if a referral is needed.

* * *

The consultation with Emily and Tony has taken a little longer than the ten minutes set aside for it and it is now twenty-five past four. When I call thirty-seven-year-old Ben in, I wonder what he has come for today. Although Ben has never been officially diagnosed, I suspect his IQ is on the lower end of normal. Ben has come to see us on a semi-regular basis with minor problems, which to us are not seen as problems at all. To Ben they are major and we always take care to treat him with respect and ensure he is taken seriously. Even if we consider the problem non-existent.

Today he appears a little downcast. What will it be today? All that was mentioned next to his name on the appointment screen was 'personal problem'.

"I've come about this problem before, but no one wants to help me with it."

When I look through Ben's notes, I notice there are four recent consultations, one with a locum two weeks ago, one with Ruth a month ago, and consultations with both of my colleagues the month before that.

"So, what can I do for you today?" Most likely next to nothing if he has come for the same reason.

"I can't seem to grow any chest hair. That can't be normal, can it? What I want is something to help me grow hair on my chest."

Yes, that was what I was afraid of. Ben has lifted his shirt up in the meantime and shows me his chest, which has little hair on it, "Why do you want to grow hair on your chest?"

Ben's eyes open wide, "How can you ask that? It's not very manly to not have a hairy chest. Not having hair on my chest makes me less of a man."

Patiently I explain that manliness has nothing to do with the amount of hair someone has or hasn't got. The success of my explanation is doubtful, "So you are not going to help me either? I should have known, you're all the same."

Even after I explain there is nothing available to help him with this problem, he remains rather angry and eventually struts out of the door, trying to slam it behind him. As the door is on a delayed closing spring, this attempt is unsuccessful. Another unhappy customer.

* * *

And if I considered Ben's consultation difficult, I am soon proven to be wrong. Fifteen-year-old Poppy attends with her mother.

"I want surgery." Is the first thing that comes out of Poppy's mouth when she enters the room.

"Now, Poppy, be patient," Mum interrupts her.

At this moment I still don't know what Poppy really is after other than surgery. What kind of surgery is still a question, although it is likely plastic surgery she is after.

Soon, Poppy makes the problem clearer, "Look at me. These breasts are horrible. The left one is tiny and the right one is huge. I have the body of an ogre. You need to refer me for surgery to have them made the same size."

Although Poppy is correct in pointing out that the breasts are different sizes, the difference is hardly noticeable and she is only fifteen. This means her body is still growing and her breasts also will. At the moment it is too early for Poppy to consider surgery, the eventual outcome would be too unpredictable.

Poppy is not a happy bunny. Even after my explanation, she tells me that my refusal to refer her is ruining her life. Actually, I did not refuse the referral, I only explained and advised. Mum tries to calm Poppy down, telling her I'm right and she should wait until she is fully grown before making such a monumental decision. When they leave, they are still arguing about this.

* * *

Five-year-old Bradley is my next patient. Today he has come with his dad. Bradley spends half the week with his mum and the other half with his dad. Tonight he will return to his mum for a few days and then return to dad again on Sunday. Although his parents are no longer together, they sorted the childcare out well between them and work together as a team where Bradley is concerned.

The reason they are here is due to a deterioration in Bradley's asthma. Over the course of today, his breathing has worsened, he is more wheezy and, although his inhalers help, he needs to use them on an hourly basis.

When I examine Bradley's chest, there are a few crackles on the right and he is very wheezy. The skin on his chest gets drawn in between his ribs a little and this is again a sign he is struggling a little. I try to test his peak flow (a breathing test), aware Bradley is likely too young to be able to perform this, and it is lower than expected for his age and height. The technique shown during this test was however poor and the result is, therefore, not accurate. When I test his oxygen levels, they are 99% and his pulse is a little fast at 106 per minute.

At the moment, I wonder if we should have Bradley admitted. When I suggest this to dad, he is adamant Bradley has been far worse than this and usually recovers quickly with antibiotics and steroids. Bradley's breathing appears to have settled a little and I agree to give Bradley antibiotics and steroids and let him go home, provided his parents will seek medical attention immediately if he does not improve or worsens overnight.

Before he leaves, I also book an appointment for the next morning to review Bradley again, "Although I officially have no appointments available tomorrow, I still want to see him again. Does ten to ten suit?"

"That sounds fine doctor. His mum can take him, she is off on Friday. Are you sure it's not too much bother?"

No, Bradley needs to be reviewed tomorrow and if creating an extra appointment before tomorrow's surgery is what is needed, I will do that. They leave, promising to re-arrange the appointment if it is not suitable after all.

* * *

At seven minutes to five Tracy comes in. She is a fifty-eight-year-old, who has suffered from left-sided sciatica for the last month. Tracy is known with a lower back problem and she is requesting something for the pain.

When I question Tracy further on her symptoms, she denies any injuries and no alarm symptoms are discovered. Tracy denies any problems with her bladder or bowel control and there is no weakness to accompany the pain. After a short examination to confirm this is simple sciatica and finding a stiffness of her left buttock, I advise her on exercises to improve her symptoms. "You can also use pain relief if needed," and after discussing the options, Tracy decides to avoid the prescription charge and buy the tablets over the counter.

"Please get back in touch if the symptoms don't improve or if they worsen."

Tracy nods and leaves the room. Time for the next patient.

* * *

When I finish writing the notes and go back to the appointment screen, I notice Tracy was the last booked appointment for today. Before continuing to the extra patients I have added, I take a quick bathroom break.

CHAPTER 26

Thursday, 5:07 pm

Ben, the forty-six-year-old man with lower backache, is the first extra patient of the afternoon. Ben phoned for a sick note this morning, which he did not require and called back later in the morning as his back pain was such he wanted to have a face-to-face consultation because of it. Or so he told the receptionist.

"Doc, I know you said I don't need a sick note, but my gaffer..., well...," Ben fidgets with a leaflet he picked up in reception, "The thing is..., he won't let me take time off unless I get a note from you. Honestly, I really need that sick note."

So, how about that backache worsening? "Can I just make sure? You are here for a sick note and not because the pain is worse? Is that correct?"

Ben nods, "Yes, it was the only way the receptionist would let me speak to you again."

"Well, here is the situation. Legally, your employer cannot ask for a doctor's note until you have been off sick for at least one week. Employers are legally bound to accept an employee's self-certificate for a duration of up to one week. Obviously, you should only use that option if you are unable to work. If your employer for some unknown reason insists on a doctor's note, there is only one option for that. I can give you a private sick note, but such a note carries a charge. A charge I believe the employer should pay, but they will often leave it to the patient to pay for it instead."

Ben nods.

"Knowing what I told you, do you want me to give you a private sick note? A note you legally do not require?"

"Well, if you put it like that. I will try my employer again and get back to you if he insists on a note from you."

"And how about your back? Is it worse, the same? Can I examine your back while you are here, so we have that to back up any notes you may require later?"

"No, really, there is no need. It is improving already. No need to bother with that. Cheerio."

Ben leaves and I wonder why people will sometimes make up things to see us.

* * *

My next patient is five-year-old Megan. When she returned from nursery at lunchtime, she had a temperature, a snotty nose and a cough. Over the last four days the cold had started, but today it is worse and mum is concerned about Megan.

"So, how has Megan been since you spoke to us?"

Mum's face lights up, "Oh, much better, thank you. Still, I figured out since I've managed to get an appointment for her, I would like Megan checking over, anyway."

Next, I ask after Megan's symptoms and mum tells me about her snotty nose and cough. She has not given her any paracetamol or ibuprofen. "Well, I really didn't want to muddy the picture for you now, did I? I assumed it would be better to see what you thought before I gave her anything."

This is not something I agree with. If you are suffering, then take something for it if you can safely do so. The pharmacist can usually advise you what to take.

When I check Megan's temperature, this is only 37.3, which is normal. Mum confirms that she does not own a thermometer and simply placed her hand against Megan's forehead to check for a fever. And she did this while Megan was upset and crying when she did not get her way.

Examination of her throat, ears, neck and chest shows no abnormalities. There is only the snotty nose as evidence of a cold, but otherwise Megan appears well. Megan also doesn't want to sit still on mother's lap. Instead, she struggles to get free so she can explore.

After advice about treatment and when to seek medical attention, Megan and her mum leave.

* * *

After two extra patients who did in hindsight not need to be seen, it is time to see thirty-four-year-old Melanie. When she makes her way into the room, her head is dipped, and she gazes at the floor. She keeps wringing her hands and appears rather uncomfortable.

"So what can I do for you today?"

Melanie looks up for a moment, "Uhm...," she glances back at her hands, "I'm pregnant."

So far, Melanie has said very little.

"And how do you feel about that?"

"Well, I don't want it," she fidgets some more, "I mean, I can't have it." Tears run down Melanie's face as she explains how she went out with friends. During the night out she had drunk more alcohol than she usually does and slept with a few men. Melanie has no idea who the father is and does not want anyone to find out she has slept around. No, Melanie is desperate to protect her reputation.

"Do you know when the first day of your last period

was?"

Melanie mentions a date six weeks ago after consulting an app on her smartphone.

Now, we discuss all the options open to Melanie, including termination, adoption, and continuing the pregnancy after all. As she is only six weeks pregnant, she still has time to ponder over the decision longer than the day she has done so far. She only found out yesterday.

Before she leaves, she accepts a card with the number for BPAS (the British Pregnancy Advisory Service) and promises to think it over a bit more. Melanie leaves with the reassurance we will still be here to support her, whatever her decision is.

* * *

Following the consultation with Melanie, the next patient on my list of emergency patients is Malcolm, a forty-three-year-old man with a painful scrotum.

"My balls have been hurting for the last two days and it is getting worse. Normally I would not mind having bigger balls, but the left one is really taking the mickey at the moment." Malcolm shuffles on his chair a little to get more comfortable, a grimace on his face.

When I ask about any injuries, he denies this.

"Do you mind if I examine you? Or would you prefer

to consult a male doctor?"

"No, I would prefer to see you. I'm here now. Anyway, I would feel even more uncomfortable if I consulted with a bloke for this."

Malcolm staggers to the couch and we pull the curtains around. He has declined the offer of a chaperone. On examination of his scrotum, the left side is swollen, and red compared to the right. It is warm to the touch, and even the slightest touch makes him wince. The problem area appears to be slightly above the left testicle, the epididymis.

All signs point towards epididymitis, an infection of the epididymis. After I explain this to Malcolm, I issue a prescription for antibiotics and ask him to return if his symptoms don't improve, dissolve or if they worsen.

Although Malcolm still grimaces with movement, he looks a little more cheerful when he leaves my room.

Now it is time for the next item on my list.

* * *

Next is the phonecall about eighty-four-year-old Leslie. Leslie's daughter Amanda has phoned with concerns about his memory. It has been a few years since I last saw him and it does not appear like he has seen anyone else at the surgery recently either. Leslie's last attendance was in October for his flu jab. I scan through his notes and can't find any mention of his memory before today.

Discussing patients with relatives is a very tricky thing. Due to confidentiality, we can not offer any information about the patient to the relative. We are, however, allowed to listen to the information the relative gives us and write this down in the notes. Not as a fact, but as hearsay. Time to brace myself for what will probably be a difficult call, relatives won't always accept that we can't give any information about their loved one, I pick up the phone and dial the daughter's number.

"Evening, is that Amanda?"

Amanda confirms this and I ask her to explain what the problem is.

"It is Dad. He has been acting rather strange lately and I'm worried about him. The problem is, I live a hundred and forty-eight miles from dad and can't just pop over whenever I like. Dad only has me; I have no brothers or sisters."

Amanda takes a breath, "Two days ago his carer phoned me. Dad had been wandering on the streets in his pyjamas at three in the morning. When the police found him, he said he was on the way to work. At three in the morning! Now I ask you. That can't be normal, right?"

One occurrence is not proof of something being wrong, however, I agree with Amanda that she has reason to worry about him a little. Instead of telling her so, I ask her if anything else has happened to worry her.

"When I last visited Dad, he seemed to think I was mum. Mum died twenty years ago, and he knows that. Dad cared for her while she died of cancer. Still, he said, 'Is that you Mary? I'm glad you're home again' and when I asked him about it, he simply brushed it under the carpet and told me I was mistaken and he had never said that."

After a brief break, Amanda continues, "Then there was the time dad left hot dogs to boil in a pan until all the fluid had evaporated. When the carer came, she found them smoking on the stove." She takes another breath, "And that time when he went shopping and not only left the door unlocked, but he left both the front door and the back door wide open."

Amanda appears to be right to worry about her dad.

"Is there any way you might be able to convince your dad to come and see us about this? Could you perhaps come with him?"

"Can't you just go and visit him. Perhaps tell him it is a routine visit to a patient of his age?"

As I explain to Amanda that it is not ethical to do so and it would also be a lie, she agrees reluctantly that I am right about that.

"Okay, I guess I should come over and bring him to the surgery one day. Do I need to phone reception or can you book the appointment for me?"

After opening the appointment screen and checking the availability over the next week, I also check to find out if she has any preference of the doctor to consult with her dad.

"Can't you see him? I mean, you now know his story." Amanda is able to visit her dad sometime next week and I again go over the appointments in the next week. None are available to be booked in advance. On Tuesday I will be on call, and it is wise to avoid a busy day like that. On Wednesday I have a normal surgery. Then on Thursday, I'm again on call and on Friday I again have a normal surgery.

"How would Wednesday suit you?"

"That sounds fine, but I can't get in early."

"Don't worry about that. There are no appointments available to book at the moment, so I will need to create one especially. Does ten to twelve sound okay?"

Amanda confirms that is perfect and I book an appointment with the nurse at half-past eleven for a blood test and ask her to bring an urine sample for her dad too. This way we can keep the number of trips to the surgery to a minimum.

"Remember to have a word with your dad about why you would like him to come to the surgery."

Amanda promises, and I put the phone back down. Ten past six already. Phew.

* * *

Before I make a start on the pile of paperwork waiting, I first take a quick bathroom break. Of course I could wait until I have finished all the paperwork, but I'm bursting already. With a bladder distracting me from my job, the progress would be slow and I would like to go home as soon as possible. It already doesn't appear likely I'll manage leaving before seven tonight.

* * *

When I return to my room, I pour another cup of tea and go through the work waiting for me; it is a lengthy list. Eighty-three tasks, one hundred and forty-eight letters, one hundred and thirty-eight results and one hundred and seventy-eight electronic prescriptions to be signed. Not to forget, the two boxes of prescriptions I have just received for signing too.

No, it definitely does not look like I will leave before

seven.

* * *

A quarter past six, I don't think I will be able to clear all the work before I leave tonight. The easiest and quickest job to get rid of is the list with electronic prescriptions. After approving their issue and entering my electronic signature, at least one box in the bottom of my screen shows zero. While the computer processed these prescriptions, I managed to sign half a box of prescriptions too. One job down, lots more to do. Already the clock shows half-past six.

* * *

The next job I tackle is the long list of tasks. Fortunately, the tasks are ordered in groups and I pick out the ones relating to prescriptions first and deal with those. I go through all the other tasks, clearing them all. A long job, but it has to be done. No one else but me to do them. When I have finally cleared the task list, it is close to seven. Will I ever get away from here and go home?

* * *

On to the next job on the list. One hundred and thirty-eight results to work through. After looking through and filing the normal results, I move on to the abnormal ones and add an appropriate comment, then send a task to the receptionists for the action to be taken.

While I act on the results, my phone beeps with a message from Martin. "Are you not ready yet?" As I glance over my desk and at my computer, I think "No, not quite ready yet" and send him a message back, "No, still busy. At least another half an hour before I can go home."

Once I have also cleared the unclassified results, I move on to the letters.

* * *

There are a lot of letters waiting for me today. That is only to be expected, Dr K was off sick this morning after all and this meant they assigned those letters to me as well as Dr P's letters. As usual, I start with the red-flagged letters to ensure I read and act on anything urgent as soon as possible. There are only twenty-five of those and I sort those out immediately. The twenty-three blue-flagged letters, all X-ray results and ultrasound results, follow. Now only the one hundred yellow-flagged, non-urgent letters remain to be read. These are next on my list.

* * *

Just after half-past seven, my eyes ache as does my head. By now I have really had enough and feel exhausted and desperate to go home. I shut down the computer, pack my bags and visit the bathroom before leaving for home. The full job may not be finished, but tomorrow is another day.

As I pick up my bags, I phone Martin, "On my way home now. Do you need anything from the shop?"

"Don't think so, maybe some crisps for the weekend?"

After I put down the phone, I make for the car, place the bags and boxes of prescriptions in the boot and drive off to go home. It has been another long day.

CHAPTER 27

Thursday, 8:00 pm

Although I don't really feel like doing the shopping tonight, I realise it will be so much more difficult tomorrow. For one, tomorrow is Friday and everyone will get their weekend groceries in. I hate being stuck in a busy shop waiting in line to pay for my shopping. The second problem is Alex will be with me tomorrow. And just like me, Alex hates shopping. No, I had better get it over and done with tonight.

During the drive home, I make a mental list of the things we need. What should we eat at the weekend? The family loves Chinese food, and the weekend is one of the few times I actually have an opportunity to cook. Yes, that will do nicely for Saturday. Hmm, maybe it will do for Sunday too. Only a slight variation needs to be made to come up with an enjoyable meal. Now I only need to decide on food for tomorrow night. Fish or mussels will do for Martin, Archie and me. The others don't like this, so I must get them fish fingers instead. Perhaps I should get croissants for the weekend, they are a bit too fiddly to bake myself, and I should also get more flour and yeast.

Before long, I take the exit to go home and drive to the supermarket. At this time of night, the shop is quiet and I get everything I need within half an hour. Only a few more minutes and I'll be home.

* * *

After parking the car on the drive, I open the door and bring in the bags. First, after greeting Martin, I take the groceries downstairs, turn on the oven and put the groceries away. Tonight we will have an easy meal, pizza. Although I will sometimes make pizza from scratch, I don't have the time to do this today. I bear it in mind for another weekend. When I make pizza myself, I use the same recipe as for bread and divide it into four pieces, which I form into pizzas. For the sauce, I use canned tomatoes, basil, oregano, garlic and chopped onion. The topping is up to whoever eats the pizza. From peas and sweet corn to salmon, prawns, mussels, scallops and other seafood to pepperoni, ham, mince. If wished, we can also add peppers, mushrooms and chillies. Cheese on top, in the oven for twenty minutes and we eat a lovely pizza to our own liking.

But tonight we go for the easy option. Fresh pizza

from the supermarket in the oven while I get changed into something more comfortable. When I return downstairs, the pizza still needs another ten minutes and I use the time to sign more prescriptions I brought home with me. Half-past eight at night is too late to get my laptop out, though. That will need to wait until tomorrow.

* * *

The oven beeps to let me know the pizza is ready. Only three prescriptions remain for signing and I finish those before moving to the oven and taking the pizza out and cutting it in half. Then I go upstairs, "Tea is ready, are you coming?"

Martin looks up from the PlayStation, "I'll be down soon."

When I return downstairs, I get a drink and take a bite of the pizza. Footsteps sound on the stairs as Martin makes his way to the kitchen. The door opens, and he joins me at the table, "Long day?"

Although that is fairly obvious, I nod. After chewing and swallowing the piece of pizza, I tell Martin about my day. "Dr K was off sick this morning, so I had a double load to deal with. All things considering, it wasn't actually too bad. If the girls wouldn't have been as supportive as they always are, it could have been much worse."

Martin nods, he knows how it is. "You shouldn't stay at work so long, though. It is not safe."

He is always very concerned about my safety and would prefer it if I would not do home visits in the evening. Where possible I will avoid this, perhaps delaying it till the next day where possible. However, this is not always a possibility. If I need to do a visit in the evening, Martin wants me to phone him before I drive to the patient and again when I leave to go home afterwards. I love how much he cares and wants to be certain I am safe.

Tonight I want to reassure Martin. "It isn't too bad, the cleaners are still there, remember. I won't stay after they leave."

Years ago I would need to stay longer. There was nothing I could do at home and all the work needed to be done at work. Sometimes we were that busy that I was still returning ring-backs at nine or half-past nine in the evening. For a moment I wonder what has changed and then I realise. In the past, we would have a fully booked surgery, twenty patients in the morning and twenty in the afternoon, and deal with the ring-backs on top of that. As we sometimes receive over fifty ring-backs in a morning and a similar number in the afternoon, it was no wonder work did not leave us with much of a private life. Fortunately, my colleagues agreed this was not a manageable workload, and we reduced the number of booked appointments when we are on call to ten in the morning and ten in the afternoon. It would be even better if we had no booked appointments at all, but the demand for appointments is too high to consider that.

For a few minutes we talk about our day at our respective work places and after putting our plates in the dishwasher and turning it on, we go upstairs. My bed is calling, it is already far past my bedtime. Tomorrow will be another early day. At least it is only half a day for me.

CHAPTER 28

Friday, 3:45 am

Friday morning already. With a yawn and a stretch, I start another day. The Fitbit buzzes me from my sleep today and I would love to stay in bed for longer. No chance of remaining in bed longer; the housework needs to be done. It is the same routine every single weekday morning. Up at a quarter to four and now it is time to get dressed. At least today is Friday. Tomorrow I will be able to have a lie-in.

Martin wraps his arm around me as I prepare to leave the bed, "I'm not letting you go," and snuggles closer to me.

It is tempting to stay in bed and I cuddle up to him a little more, "Are you sure? There won't be any fresh bread if you don't let me get up."

Martin pulls me a little closer and kisses my back, "Okay, then." After letting go of me, he gently pushes my backside towards the edge, "Up you go. Can't do without fresh bread now, can we?"

There is a twinkle in his eyes when I turn around to

kiss Martin and get up. He still has over an hour left before he needs to get up. Still, it's an early start for him again today too. On Monday and Friday morning Martin leaves at half-past five in the morning.

* * *

When I am dressed, I enter the kitchen and start preparing the dough. As every day, I unpack the dishwasher and clean the worktops while waiting for the dough to rest. The table is set for breakfast and I knead the dough for the second time and leave it to rest again. Next, I make my way to the utility room to gather the laundry. It is time to do the folding and ironing again. After ten minutes I place the dough on the worktop and form the bread rolls, then leave them to rest for a few minutes while I return to the ironing. In the background the television shows 'Hard Talk' and I now place the bread rolls in the oven for twenty minutes, while returning to the ironing once more.

At ten to five, I take them out of the oven, the ironing now finished, and put them to the side to cool a little while I put the ironing board and iron away again. The weather forecast comes on and I switch on the kettle to prepare coffee for Martin. He will get up any minute now and if I make his coffee now, it will cool enough to drink before he leaves for work.

Next, I prepare the lunches for everyone, eat a bread roll for breakfast and watch the early morning programme on TV. Bread tastes so much nicer when it is freshly baked.

The kitchen door opens, "Morning, did you sleep well?" I move over to Martin and kiss him good morning with a hug. Together we take in the news and before long the weather forecast comes on again. This is the signal it's time for Martin to leave for work, nearly half-past five already.

* * *

Once Martin has left, I return to the kitchen to get a bucket and a mop and return upstairs to clean the bathrooms. The usual race against time starts again. When the bathrooms are clean twenty minutes later, I clean the kitchen floor, the washing machine and the bin, taking the bin bag to the wheelie bin in the garage. When I return and have put a fresh bin bag in the bin, I load up the washing machine and switch it on.

A quick look at the clock tells me it is six. It is time to move on to the next job.

* * *

After getting the vacuum cleaner, I vacuum the entire house while realising this will upset my daughter again no end. Leaving it until the afternoon is not an option. Although I tried in the past, I know I don't have the energy then and it will simply be left instead. Archie and Adam also arrive in the kitchen for their breakfast and I start the job upstairs. That way I can also collect any crumbs they leave after their breakfast.

* * *

Once the vacuuming is done, it is already close to seven. Amy has also eaten her breakfast, she again scolded me for waking her on the way down, and now I have a quick shower before work and the school run. Around half-past seven I'm ready for the day ahead and on my way downstairs with the laundry, I wake up Alex for his breakfast, "Morning, sweetheart. Are you awake yet? It's time to get up."
A sleepy head emerges from the bedcovers as he throws the covers off and gets ready for his breakfast.

* * *

Now it is time to get my laptop out again and get some work out of the way. This morning I will be on call. It is rather tricky as I won't be able to get into work until around half-past nine due to the school run this morning. Still, I will be on call from eight. Until I leave for the school run, I will be available on the laptop and my mobile phone. The receptionists are fully aware I will not answer any calls while driving unless I can safely pull over or answer hands-free. Unfortunately, the hands-free set which comes with the phone is not great and often will fall from my ear. Generally, it is safer to not answer at all. The girls know this and if anything happens which can't wait until I'm at the surgery, they will seek help from one of my colleagues instead.

For now, I work through the results added during the night. Then I sign any prescriptions already added by a receptionist this morning and clear a few more of the letters I did not have a chance to read last night. Before long it is eight. As I don't need to leave yet, I continue to observe the appointment list for today.

Shortly after eight, the ring-backs start to arrive. I try to clear some of those before I even leave the house.

* * *

Now it's time to start. The first ring-back is from two-year-old Jack's mum. She is concerned Jack may have tonsillitis and insists he should see a doctor today. Okay, this seems fair enough. I send a task to the receptionists to invite Jack for a sit and wait appointment at twenty to twelve.

* * *

The second ring-back is from forty-three-year-old Henry. Henry complains of pain in his groin and would like to have an appointment today. A task is on its way to the receptionists to offer an appointment at ten to twelve.

* * *

Twelve-year-old Joseph suffers from a sore throat and grandma has phoned to request an appointment. The task to invite him for a sit and wait appointment at twelve is soon on its way to the receptionists too.

* * *

The fourth ring-back on the screen is for thirty-four-year-old Amelia, who stood on a rusty nail last night and would like to see us about this. Amelia is unsure if part of the nail was left in her foot. This is not something we can sort out and I send a task to the receptionists to advise Amelia to attend A&E with this instead. If any part of the rusty nail remains embedded in Amelia's foot, A&E will be able to look into and treat this much better. They also have access to x-ray and will receive the results of any x-ray within minutes. For any x-rays we request, it can take up to two weeks for the results to reach us.

* * *

Amelia was the last ring-back for now. It is ten past eight and time to get ready to leave. After closing down the laptop and returning it to its bag, I grab my bags and take them with me upstairs, leaving them at the front door. On my way to the bathroom, I enter Alex's room, "Time to get ready to leave." At least he is dressed in his school uniform already, Alex only needs to put his shoes on and he will be ready to leave.

In the bathroom, I use the toilet, then apply eyeshadow and lipstick. Soon I am also ready to leave and meet Alex at the front door. Twenty past eight; we need to go.

CHAPTER 29

Friday, 8:40 am

Alex and I arrive at school around twenty to nine. School doesn't start until nine and I hope the teachers will arrive soon. As soon as the first teacher arrives on the playground and I'm certain there is supervision present, I turn towards Alex, "I'll be off now, see you this afternoon." I would love to kiss him goodbye, but Alex feels too old for that now. "Not in front of my friends, mum!"

Then I leave to return to the car and drive to work. The rush hour has already cleared by now, and the journey only takes thirty minutes. During the drive, my thoughts drift to the early that morning when Martin wouldn't let me get out of bed. I really have lucked out with that guy and I love him to bits. Such a pity too I couldn't stay in bed for longer and snuggle up to him some more. We'll have to make up for that this weekend.

* * *

When I arrive at the surgery, the gate is open already as expected. After all, it is twenty past nine already and the doors open at eight. Next, I park the car, noticing Dr K has used the slot I usually use, get out, grab my bags and let myself in through the back door. I drop off the signed prescriptions at reception and make for my room. There I put my bags away safely, turn on the computer and pour myself a cup of tea while waiting for the computer to start up. It's time to get ready for the morning of appointments and ring-backs ahead.

* * *

After logging onto Windows and starting the clinical system, I pay a visit to the bathroom before logging onto the clinical system. No reason to leave personal details of patients available for anyone who would enter my room.

* * *

When I return to my room, another seven ring-backs have been added since I logged off from the laptop earlier. The fourth ring-back is also back on the list again. This was the lady who stood on a nail last night. Why would she ring-back after the advice I gave?

CHAPTER 30

Friday, 9:35 am

Amelia is not happy with the advice I gave her to go to A&E and wants to see someone at the surgery before she will go there. Although I doubt this is appropriate, I look at the appointment list for Ruth, our nurse, and notice she has one appointment available today. After blocking that appointment and stating this one is intended for Amelia, I send a task to the receptionists to offer her that one. If Amelia feels this is inconvenient, she can go to A&E instead. I still believe she should go there, anyway.

* * *

The fifth ring-back of today is for seventy-six-year-old Mabel, who complains of a swollen and painful big toe. Mabel would like to see a doctor today about this. In response to her request, I send a task to the receptionists to offer her an appointment at ten past twelve. The list of extras is growing steadily.

* * *

The next ring-back on my list is from thirty-four-year-old Sally, who requests the morning-after pill. At twenty to ten, I pick up the phone and call her.

"Last night I had sex with my partner and the condom broke. Can I have the morning-after pill please?"

After inquiring further, I learn Sally is not on any other contraception than condoms. Neither has she any reasons why she should not use the morning-after pill, "A prescription will be available to pick up from reception in the next few minutes. You can pick this up any time before we close at six. Take the tablet as soon as possible for best efficacy. If your period is any different from what you are used to or if it is late, do a pregnancy test and make sure. No method of contraception works 100%," I take a breath, "I would also advise you to book an appointment with a nurse or doctor to discuss other methods of contraception which are more reliable than condoms. Perhaps you would like to consider one of the longer acting forms like the coil or the implant. A leaflet about these options will be included with your prescription."

"Thanks, doctor, that is great. I'll make that appointment when I come to pick my prescription up."

I also make a mention in her notes of the advice given about long-acting contraception to fulfil the requirements of the Quality and Outcomes Framework (QOF) and move on to the next problem on the list.

* * *

The next ring-back is an easy one to solve. Twenty-eight-year-old Darren wants to see me to treat a dental abscess. As a General Practitioner, dental abscesses do not fall under my field of expertise and I, therefore, can't treat them. This is a problem for which Darren will need to consult the dentist instead, and I send a task to the receptionists to ask them to inform him of this. I am certain the receptionist already told him this, but Darren probably wanted a doctor to confirm this.

* * *

The eighth ring-back is from fifty-six-year-old Victor, who has a painful lump down below. Victor asks to see a doctor today. This problem will need an examination, and I send a task to invite him for twenty past twelve.

* * *

Nearly ten to ten. The next ring-back is from seventy-two-year-old Patricia, who believes she may have a chest infection. She has a cough and brings up green phlegm. Patricia's request for an appointment is honoured with a task to the receptionists to invite her for a half-past twelve sit-and-wait appointment.

* * *

Now I move on to the tenth ring-back. Seven-year-old Jerome has a sore finger and mum believes it is infected. An offer for a twenty to one sit-and-wait appointment leaves as a task to the receptionists. This should also be convenient for Jerome, as he should be on his lunch break at that time.

* * *

The next ring-back is from a patient who is requesting the results from a cholesterol test. Although the results have arrived, my colleague has not yet had a chance to act on it. The request from the receptionist is if I could look at the result instead so we can inform Brian as she already told him the result has arrived. Why did she do that? Now Brian wants to receive the results now instead of waiting for the doctor to assess the result first. It would have been much better to tell him the result was still awaited.

When I glance through his notes, there is no obvious

reason documented why the test was done. The cholesterol level is good at 3.8. Again, I go through his notes and on his repeat list I notice Brian is on a cholesterol tablet. Aha, it must be a part of the medication review. In response, I file the result and send the task to the receptionists to inform Brian that the cholesterol tablet seems to be working well, to continue to take this as the cholesterol looks good at 3.8.

I should speak with Patricia again about letting patients know a test result has arrived. This places us in a rather awkward spot where we need to assess a result when something more urgent might wait for us.

* * *

My patient from yesterday has arrived for his review. Although more ring-backs are present on my screen, it is time to call Bradley in first. As you may remember, Bradley is the five-year-old boy who attended with his dad last night. When I examined Bradley last night, his chest was wheezy, and he had some problems with his breathing as well as a chest infection. Only after dad promised to seek medical attention if Bradley did not improve or if he got worse overnight, did I allow him to go home rather than arrange an admission. Today I need to find out if the antibiotics and steroids I gave

Bradley last night have improved his symptoms.

At six to ten Bradley trails in with his mum, "See, I told you it was this room," Bradley pulls his mum into the room. Next, he starts running around the room, playing 'aeroplane'. He appears to be a lot better than yesterday.

"So, how has Bradley been since yesterday?"

Mum tears her eyes from Bradley to look at me, "Much better, he last used his inhaler about three hours ago."

That indeed sounds much better. He needed it hourly yesterday. When I listen to his chest, it is far less wheezy and the crackles appear to be less too. "Great, it appears Bradley is getting better. Continue to give him the medication until it runs out and if his symptoms worsen or don't improve further, then please come back to have him examined again."

A happy mum and a much healthier seeming Bradley leave the room.

* * *

Now I turn my attention to the twelfth ring-back of the morning. The nursing home requests a home visit for ninety-six-year-old William, who has a nasty cough. Will I be able to visit William? The morning already is busy and I need to bear in mind I'll need to pick up Alex from school at half-past three. There is no choice, I will have to try. Mind made up, I send a task to the receptionists I will attempt to visit at lunchtime and let them know if anything happens to make this impossible.

* * *

By now it is two minutes past ten, and my first patient has arrived. Although there are more ring-backs waiting, the booked patients need to come first for now. None of the ring-backs has any message with them to inform me they are urgent.

Five-year-old Mollie comes in with her mum, "School told me to see you. Mollie has head lice and needs something for it."

I examine Mollie's head, and some head lice and nits are visible. Although medication is available to treat this, lotions mainly, they no longer work adequately for it. Over the years, the head lice have become insensitive to the treatment, and this means the old-fashioned treatment of using conditioner and a nit-comb works the best. When I inform mum of this, she is not very impressed. Grudgingly she makes her way out again after my advice to consult a pharmacist if there is no improvement after a week. The pharmacist also runs a minor illness clinic and can prescribe for this problem if appropriate.

* * *

Next on the appointment list today is thirty-seven-year-old Robert, who comes to request plastic surgery on the NHS (National Health Service). Robert's problem is that his penis is too small and he can't satisfy women. Or so previous girlfriends have led him to believe. Robert wants me to examine him for this problem, something which makes me feel a little uncomfortable. There is always a risk Robert will turn this into a complaint about inappropriate examination at a later stage. Still, Robert is in distress and needs his problem addressing. As a compromise, I agree with him to ask someone to act as a chaperone and a receptionist stands in the room while I examine Robert.

No abnormalities show themselves today. I cannot examine the maximum size of Robert's penis. That would be inappropriate without a doubt. After reassuring him everything appears to be normal and size is not really important, he still insists on referral.

Now it is time to talk to him about the procedure he requests. This is not available on the NHS and unlikely to be successful. What Robert needs is something he will not agree to. Psychological support and consulting with a counsellor would benefit him more. It would also be required if he ever was to be referred.

Disappointed with the outcome, Robert leaves. Sometimes people bring problems we can't solve. However hard we try. Hopefully Robert is more lucky with his next girlfriend. What an awful thing to say to someone. He has obviously not met the right person yet.

* * *

Still mulling over Robert's problem, I close his notes and return to the appointment screen. Even more ring-backs arrived and as a result, the stress levels are building. How am I going to get through all the work before leaving to pick Alex up?

The next patient is fifty-three-year-old Russell, a type two diabetic. Russell has noticed a slightly red area on his left foot and wonders if this is an ulcer.

When I examine his feet, they both are absolutely fine, no redness is visible and there is no sign of an ulcer.

After complimenting Russell on his vigilance and coming to have his feet checked, I reiterate advice previously given about foot care and seeking medical attention if he finds any signs of injury. I also ask him to return if the symptoms don't improve.

While I write in Russell's notes, an instant message

from Ruth pops up, "Can you have a look at a patient with me, please?" I finish writing the notes and leave my room.

* * *

With Ruth is forty-three-year-old Helen, who has a rash down below, or in other words, in her private area. The area appears red, and the skin is peeling slightly while an off-white discharge is visible at the entry of her vagina. This looks most like thrush and I advise Ruth to take swabs to exclude other infections and to treat this as vaginal thrush in the meantime. Armed with a prescription for Canesten cream and pessary, Helen seems happier, if still uncomfortable.

"Don't forget to come back if the rash does not settle down."

Helen nods and a cheeky grin appears on her face, "Even though I'm not Arnold Schwarzenegger, I'll be back. But only if the rash doesn't improve."

* * *

When I return to my room, I decide to check a few more ring-backs before calling in the next patient on my list.

The thirteenth ring-back is a prescription request

from the district nurse. A housebound patient needs cream for his dry legs and I issue the requested prescription and send a task to inform the receptionists of this.

* * *

The next ring-back is also from the district nurse. This time a prescription request for some catheter bags and equipment. After I have completed this request, issued the prescription and informed the receptionists, I continue to the next problem.

I notice fifty-three prescriptions are waiting to be signed electronically and I get rid of those first. Fifty-three fewer prescriptions to deal with before home time.

* * *

Now it is time to call in my fourth patient. Thirty-three-year-old Samantha experimented with dyeing her hair last week. She got together with some friends and each helped the others to give their hair a different colour. Over the last week, Samantha has suffered with a red, angry rash on her forehead, which is now peeling. It burns and itches and today is the first day she dared to leave the house.

When I examine the skin on Samantha's forehead, an obvious eczematous rash is present, most likely an allergic reaction to the hair dye.

"But it can't be. The box stated it was a hypo-allergenic formula."

Even if the box made that claim, it still does not mean she can't have an allergic reaction to the ingredients, "I would still recommend not to use this again. Perhaps it is even better to avoid any hair dyes in the future."

Samantha's expression turns darker. She is not a happy bunny. "This was only a bit of fun."

After giving her a mild steroid cream to help with the rash, Samantha leaves. Even a bit of fun can turn into not much fun at all.

* * *

Twenty-three-year-old Elizabeth is my next patient. She has come for a pill check. During the consultation Elizabeth tells me she experiences no problems with the pill, remembers to take it on time and she does not smoke. Elizabeth's weight is stable and normal and there is no reason she can't continue with the pill.

While we discuss longer-acting forms of contraception, the phone rings.

"Sorry to disturb you, Dr Ellen. I have the district

nurse on the line. Could she have a word with you please, she tells me it's urgent?"

Libby puts the call through, "Morning, this is Dr Ellen, can you hang on for a brief moment while I finish the consultation? Should not be long at all."

I turn the phone on mute and return to Elizabeth, explaining about the other forms of contraception and within a minute she leaves, a prescription for her preferred pill in hand. Now it is time to pay attention to what the district nurse has to tell me.

* * *

After turning the phone back to normal, I ask the district nurse what I can help her with.

"I'm sorry to disturb you. Do you know Trevor? Trevor is a fifty-eight-year-old man with terminal bowel cancer. His pain relief is no longer sufficient and I would like you to visit him to assess what we need to do next. The other problem is that Trevor has not been seen for the last two weeks by a doctor and I think he may not last the weekend. Can you please visit Trevor and sort his medication out?"

With Trevor, I definitely have no choice. Trevor needs to have a visit before the weekend. The problem is how busy the on-call is already and I will need to get to school in time for Alex. After explaining this problem to the district nurse, we decide the changes in medication that are required. I issue a prescription for this medication and an updated syringe-driver instruction form. With a promise to visit Trevor on my way home, we end the call.

* * *

With the interruptions to my surgery, I now run fifteen minutes behind schedule. Fortunately, my next patient is forty-six-year-old Jennifer. Jennifer shows me an itchy rash on her feet, tiny blisters and peeling skin with a white appearance to the skin. After explaining to Jennifer she suffers from Athlete's foot and handing her a prescription for Canesten cream, Jennifer leaves. Her problem only took five minutes and now I'm only ten minutes behind.

* * *

Now, I quickly check the next ring-back, the sixteenth for today. Thirty-four-year-old Emily complains of symptoms of a urine infection and requests antibiotics to treat this. Instead of taking Emily's word as gospel, I send a task to request a urine sample to investigate her symptoms further.

* * *

Twelve past eleven already. The pressure is getting to me and my face burns while my chest feels heavy. How can I speed up my work and still give the patients all the attention they deserve and not miss anything?

The next patient is fifty-six-year-old Violet, "It's this lump, doctor. Should I be worried about it?" Apparently Violet read in a magazine about a woman with a lump on her leg and this turned out to be cancer.

"How long have you had the lump for?"

Violet's expression turns thoughtful, "Uhm..., not sure. You see, the lump has been present for as long as I can remember."

When I ask her if it has changed at all, Violet ponders on this for a moment, "No, not really."

Now I examine the lump which is smooth, round and a little flexible. It looks like a lipoma, a fatty lump.

"No, you don't need to worry about this lump, it is a local collection of fatty tissue and is absolutely innocent."

Violet wants to know if we need to remove it and again I reassure her there is no need to do so. The entire consultation only takes five minutes, and I have caught up a little more.

* * *

Before seeing the last two patients who are booked for this morning's surgery, I contact the next ring-back.

Fifty-six-year-old Valerie came to see me last week. At the time she complained of muscle aches and Valerie was convinced this meant she suffered from rheumatoid arthritis. The consultation had been particularly difficult as she was convinced of the truth in her statements and also convinced I did everything in my power to stop her from confirming the truth. In reality, I only tried to reassure her that her symptoms did not fit with a diagnosis of rheumatoid arthritis, which centres around the joints and not the muscles, and wanted to avoid exposing Valerie to tests she did not require.

Once I had convinced her of the fact that I was willing to organise blood test for her and gave her a form to enable Valerie to do so, she settled down and left happier than before, but still convinced she suffered from rheumatoid arthritis. One of her friends even told me later in the week, "You saw my friend Valerie two days ago, didn't you?" Obviously, I was unable to confirm this. "Valerie has rheumatoid arthritis, she tells me. You confirmed that for her."

All I could do was to mumble I couldn't remember and move on to the problem her friend had come with.

Today Valerie has rung to find out the results of her

blood tests and requesting a ring-back so I can explain the results. As expected, the blood tests were completely normal.

"Valerie? Morning, this is Dr Ellen." After one more glance at the results, I continue. "You wanted to know the results of your blood test." Valerie makes confirming noises. "Well, the blood tests have come back entirely normal. This means there is no sign of rheumatoid arthritis, just like we discussed last week. So, that is good news."

She asks me why her muscles are aching if it is not rheumatoid arthritis and when I ask her how they currently are, she tells me the muscles feel okay again now.

"In that case it appears it was only a simple muscle ache after all." I am still not convinced Valerie believes me. Even if the pain had now disappeared.

* * *

At the moment it is twenty past eleven and I'm running ten minutes behind schedule. Not bad considering the load on my desk again today. Hopefully, I can maintain control and finish surgery on time.

My next patient is fifty-eight-year-old Oliver, who has found a lump in his right groin. He has noticed the lump on and off for a few months; it appeared after lifting something heavy. The lump does not cause Oliver any pain or discomfort, but he has noted it is occasionally larger. After gaining his consent to examine him, I ask him to remain standing. I suspect Oliver has an inguinal hernia (a hernia in his groin) and if Oliver would lie down this would likely disappear.

A small lump is palpable and when I ask Oliver to cough, the lump gets larger. Now the diagnosis is confirmed, I explain to Oliver what the problem is and what we should do next. With the advice to seek medical attention if it becomes painful or if he can't push it back in, I offer to refer Oliver for a surgical opinion. In most cases, inguinal hernia operations are day cases. Oliver agrees, and I hand him a paper to book an appointment at reception. Our file room assistant books the appointment through the choose and book system directly at the hospital and Oliver will know when he will be seen at the hospital for this problem before he leaves the surgery.

As soon as the door closes behind Oliver, I write the letter to the specialist to explain his problem, the finding, any medical history of importance and any allergies. Then it is time to move on to the last booked patient of today.

* * *

Only one more patient remains. That is, of the list of patients who were booked into existing appointments. The rest of today's list consists of ring-backs and emergency patients.

Sixty-three-year-old Jeffrey saunters in and glances around him hesitantly.

"Come in and have a seat," I force a welcoming smile on my face.

A red flush colours his cheeks, "You're a female."

I can't deny that, "That is right. Did you want to see a male doctor instead?"

"Well, I'm here now, anyway."

Jeffrey tells me about his embarrassing problem, "My foreskin is that tight if I go for a wee, everything squirts everywhere. It's time I saw someone about it. Sometimes the foreskin even swells up like a balloon before I can finally urinate."

After an examination confirms an excessively tight foreskin or phimosis as it is known in the medical world, we agree I will refer Jeffrey to the urology department for assessment and treatment. At Jeffrey's age, this is not a pleasant operation. I suspect it is not at any age, but at least young children will have no memory of it. Forewarned about this, Jeffrey leaves my room, a form to book a choose and book appointment in his hand.

While I write the referral letter, another message from Ruth to check a patient with her pops up on my screen.

* * *

Ruth turns to me as I enter her room, "Ah, thank you for coming, doctor. This is eighty-two-year-old Elsie. A carer noticed a mole on her back and I would like you to give your opinion on it."

When I examine the mole, it is dark but has different shades of brown within the mole. The mole is irregularly shaped and has all the appearances of a melanoma; skin cancer.

"Well, Elsie, we will need to have that checked over at the hospital." While I talk to Elsie and explain about my suspicions taking care not to scare her too much, I fill in the referral form for suspected skin cancer. After printing it off and handing it to the carer who has come with her, I ask them to take the form to reception, where an appointment can be booked for the hospital. This should be an appointment within the next two weeks. I advise them to contact the surgery if the appointment does not fall within the next two weeks.

CHAPTER 31

Friday, 11:45 am

It is a quarter to twelve when I return to my room and focus my attention on the eighteenth ring-back of today. Sixty-two-year-old Beverley wants to discuss her cholesterol tablets.

"Have you seen the news this week, doctor? Cholesterol tablets are bad for us, the tablets increase the blood sugar levels and cause diabetes. I would like to stop taking them if they give me diabetes." Beverley's agitated voice betrays her concerns.

After reassuring her she can stop the cholesterol tablets if she wishes, a deep sigh escapes from Beverley. Next, I explain the evidence surrounding this news and once she finds out her risks of a heart attack or stroke without the tablets is higher than the risk of diabetes while taking them, Beverley decides she wants to continue the statins after all.

Then I offer further reassurance, "Your annual blood test includes your sugar level as standard. So far there is no sign of diabetes and we will continue to monitor that."

Beverley is happy with the explanations and we end the call.

* * *

The next ring-back is from the grandma of three-year-old Aidan. Nursery sent him home this morning with a cough, temperature and discharging eye. Staff at the nursery believe he has conjunctivitis and is contagious to the other children in their care. Soon a task to invite him for a sit-and-wait appointment at ten to one is on the way to the receptionists.

* * *

Jack, the two-year-old boy with possible tonsillitis has also arrived, and he has been waiting for nearly a quarter of an hour The rest of the ring-backs will need to wait while I call Jack in.

Mum bursts into the room, Jack in tow, "Thank you so much for seeing Jack, I have been so worried about him." Mum's eyes are wide as saucers and her hands shake. When I look at Jack, he does not appear as unwell as mum's appearance suggests. I ask mum about his symptoms and words spew from her mouth, "Jack is very unwell, his tonsils are huge and red and he feels so hot. He is burning up and really worries me."

At that moment, Jack is struggling to get away from her to explore the room. When I ask her if she checked his temperature, she seems disbelieving, as though that is the weirdest question to ask, "Jack has a fever, you can tell simply by touching his forehead. Here, try for yourself if you don't believe me."

I take that as a 'no' and examine the patient instead. Jack's temperature is normal at 37.2 and mum blurts out, "Oh, it must have come down after I gave him paracetamol earlier." When I ask when Jack last had paracetamol, this turns out to be last night. As paracetamol only works for about four or six hours at the most, this will not have affected Jack's current temperature. The glands in his neck are normal and although the tonsils are slightly red, there are no white spots on them and they are not really enlarged either. Jack's ears and chest are fine too and I reassure mum this is only a variation of normal and with his temperature at a normal level at the moment too, Jack needs no further treatment than monitoring him. I give her the usual advice to seek further medical attention if his symptoms worsen or don't improve and they leave and I am not convinced mum believes me.

* * *

The next emergency is Henry, a forty-three-year-old man who complains about groin pain. When he walks in, he does so with a slight limp. Henry sits down and tells me his story, "This groin has been causing me trouble for the last two days. I love playing football and I'm also kicking a ball with the lads. When I was playing with the kids two days ago, I slipped and felt something twist in my right hip. This has been hurting since."

On examination, there is not much to be found. There is no sign of a hernia and the tendons in his right groin are tender to the touch. After explaining he suffers from a groin strain, Henry leaves again, reassured. Henry knows to return if his symptoms don't settle or worsen.

* * *

Now it is time to call in twelve-year-old Joseph, the boy with a sore throat.

Joseph shoots in ahead of a male adult, "Morning doctor, I'm Joseph's grandad." He holds out his hand for me to shake, "Joseph lives with his grandma and me as his mum is in no position to look after him. Our daughter is a drug addict, you see, and we have a residential order for Joseph to live with us."

Ah, I remember, Joseph's dad died a few years ago of a drug overdose and Joseph has lived with his grandparents more or less since birth.

When I enquire after Joseph's symptoms, grandad tells me that for the last three days, Joseph has complained of a sore throat and this has gradually worsened over the last few days.

On examination, the glands in his neck are swollen, as are his tonsils. The tonsils have white spots covering them and his temperature is 38.4. After diagnosing Joseph with tonsillitis, I prescribe antibiotics and advise a review if his symptoms worsen or don't improve.

* * *

The fifth extra patient today is seventy-six-year-old Mabel with her painful big toe. I have caught up a little and now only run four minutes behind schedule. The pressure is still on as there are still a lot of ring-backs waiting, two visits and paperwork to be done before I can leave to pick up Alex.

Mabel shows me her right big toe, which is swollen, red and hot to the touch. She is not keen for me to touch the toe either. The swelling is worst at the ball of her foot and as she has had no injury to the toe, it is most likely Mabel suffers from gout.

"Have you heard of gout?" Mabel nods. "They also call it the rich man's disease as in the olden days, the lords of the manor would sometimes be affected by this. If you go to castles and manors, you still often see the lord of the manor with a foot on a stool and a bandage around his big toe. That was gout. Gout is caused by uric acid crystals which collect in a joint, irritate the joint and then cause inflammation of the joint. That is most likely what happened to your toe." Mabel takes in my words and nods her understanding so far. "To treat this, we need to give you something to help with the pain and the inflammation. We will also need to arrange for a blood test to confirm this is indeed gout. If we confirm this is gout, we can consider giving you medication to decrease the levels of uric acid in the blood and therefore the risk of getting another attack."

"Can't you give me that already?"

Unfortunately it does not quite work that way, "If we give you that treatment already, it will lower the uric acid levels in the blood, but it will also push it to go into the joint instead and make the attack worse. No, we will need to wait until the attack has gone, at which time the uric acid moves out of the joints again and we can then confirm if this is or is not gout. If we treat the uric acid after that, this should help to reduce the number of attacks you would suffer."

Was I making this clear or was it only getting more confusing? Mabel nodded, and I hoped this meant she understood what I had told her.

"Now, there are a few things you can do to help. There is some evidence eating cherries reduces the uric acid levels. Red meat, wine, and other forms of alcohol and cheese are known to increase the levels, so you may wish to reduce the intake of those. Sometimes attacks are provoked by slight trauma, like stubbing your toe. Any questions?"

Mabel seems to understand what I have told her, "Thomas also suffers from gout, I think the doctor told him the same thing a few years ago."

Thomas is Mabel's husband of over fifty years. That explains why she did not appear to be more confused by my explanation. I hand Mabel a prescription and the request for blood tests and ask her to return to discuss the results.

* * *

While I wait for the next patient to come in, I move to the electronic prescription screen, highlight ten prescriptions and authorise and sign them. There are another one hundred and thirty waiting, but Victor will enter the room any moment now. Victor is the fifty-six-year-old man complaining of a painful lump down below.

"Thank you for seeing me," Victor sits on one cheek of his buttocks and leans forward, "The problem, is, I have this lump on my lower back, just north of my anus and it is really painful. Can you check it out and help me with it, please?"

As always, I offer Victor a chaperone which he declines, "I'm already embarassed enough to have to drop my pants, I don't want two people to see what's hiding underneath them."

We move to the examination couch and Victor shows me the offending lump. He has an abscess on his tailbone and it seems furiously red.

"The problem is an abscess. We can treat this with antibiotics. However, if the symptoms don't improve or if they worsen, you will need to come back. In that case, we will need to assess it again and it may require a referral for incision at the hospital at that time." The official term for this procedure is incision (cut) and drainage.

Victor leaves with a prescription for antibiotics, a promise he will return if needed, and I advise him to buy one of those rings children use to learn to swim. Sitting on one of those will relieve the pressure on the abscess and help Victor to be more comfortable.

* * *

Before I continue with the next emergency patient waiting for me, I read through the notes of the next ring-back. Forty-six-year-old Sandra was recently prescribed ramipril for her blood pressure. Over the last few days she has been plagued with a tickly cough and after reading the leaflet with the medication, she has found this to be a known side-effect. Sandra wants to know if she needs to stop the medication.

Usually, this is not a reason to stop the medication. Instead, I send a task to the receptionists to advise Sandra to continue taking the medication for the moment and to make a routine appointment to discuss this matter with a doctor. This is a known side-effect, but unless she has problems of discoloured phlegm, a temperature or breathlessness, we can assess this problem in a routine appointment.

* * *

The twenty-first ring-back of today is from eighty-year-old Thomas. He has phoned the surgery at the advice of 111. 111 is a service provided to give patients advice on medical problems. In the past, a similar service was called NHS Direct. Basically, if you need medical advice and it is not a real emergency where an ambulance needs to be called, you ring 111 to speak to a medical professional who will tell whether you can ignore the symptoms, need to call for an ambulance, speak with your doctor urgently or book a routine appointment. Our experience has not been brilliant, but 111 provides a service when we are overstretched.

When Thomas spoke to 111, he asked for advice on a rash he has suffered with for the last eight weeks. Both arms are itchy and dry, red, and the rash is a little raised. Thomas likens it to dry skin. Although he has a moisturiser at home and is happy to try this, 111 have told him he needs to consult a doctor today. From the description Thomas has provided, the problem appears to be eczema, and the moisturiser seems an excellent idea. However, with the advice we need to see him today, I would be stupid to ignore this. Although I realise this appointment will most likely be a waste of time both for Thomas and for myself, I send a task to the receptionists to invite him for a sit-and-wait appointment at one.

* * *

Nearly twenty to one; I need to hurry. Next is seventy-two-year-old Patricia, who phoned about a suspected chest infection.

"Thank you for seeing me, I'm not normally ill but three days ago I started coughing, and it hasn't stopped since. I'm bringing up this horrible green gunk and I am hot one moment and freezing the next."

When I ask Patricia if she has any breathlessness, she shakes her head, "No, only when I'm stuck in one of those coughing fits but otherwise I'm fine."

Patricia is flushed and shivers. Her temperature at the moment is 38.3, raised but not a fever. After clipping the oximeter (oxygen measuring tool) to Patricia's finger, the levels are 98%, normal. Not surprisingly, her pulse is high at ninety-six beats per minute. Crackles can be heard on the left side of her lower chest; this confirms a chest infection. After prescribing antibiotics and advising Patricia to return if there is no improvement or if she gets worse, she makes her way out of my room again.

* * *

Next, Jerome slinks in with his mum. A sore finger in this seven-year-old was the reason for mum to contact the surgery. It is nearly ten to one although the appointment offered was for twenty to one. This was, however, a sit-and-wait appointment.

Mum appears harassed and angry, "About time as well! We have been waiting for half an hour for you to call us in." Had she been a little girl I would expect her to stamp her feet. She resembled a girl in the middle of a temper tantrum.

"My apologies, I'm sorry for your wait. However, Jerome was offered an appointment which did not exist and was created especially for him. You will also have been told that this was a sit-and-wait appointment, and that is exactly what it means. The patient sits and waits until the doctor is able to see him. Although I'm sorry to be behind on schedule and you have had to wait, this is not unexpected during the time I am on call and running only ten minutes behind is actually quite good."

I should not argue with mum over this, but she really got under my skin, "But let's look at Jerome's finger, shall we?" Next I face Jerome, "Which finger is the poorly one?"

Jerome pulls his fingers out of his mouth and points to his right middle finger. The nails are minuscule and give the impression of bitten nails. Around the nail bed of this finger, this finger is swollen, red and there is a pussy discharge. This is called a whitlow or an infection of the soft tissue of the finger.

"Do you bite your nails?" I place what I hope is a

reassuring smile on my face.

Jerome shuffles his feet, looks down and nods.

"That is not a good idea, is it?"

He shakes his head.

"If you bite your nails, this can happen. Would you like me to give you something to make it better?"

Jerome looks up and nods his head. After explaining to mum what has happened, she seems to have calmed down a little, I give them a prescription for antibiotics to treat this and advise to return if the problem worsens or doesn't improve.

On the way out, I can hear mum tell Jerome, "See, I told you, this doctor is nice."

That was a close one. I really shouldn't have lost my patience with her.

* * *

The end of today's surgery is in sight. Only three more ring-backs on the list, two extras awaited and several urine samples. Before calling the next patient in, I read the next ring-back. This one is from twenty-seven-year-old Amy, who has received an invitation for a cervical smear. She has phoned to ask if she should have a smear at the moment. Amy is pregnant with her second child and wonders if she should have a smear while pregnant. She is right to query this; we do not advise smears during pregnancy.

The problem is easily solved; I send a task to the receptionists to advise Amy to delay the smear until three months after the birth.

After doing this, I move to the electronic prescription screen, highlight twenty-five of the prescriptions, authorise and sign them, then call for the next patient.

* * *

The next patient is three-year-old Aidan. Grandma contacted us about his cough, temperature and gunky eye and she is with Aidan now. He seems active and friendly. That friendly, he almost climbs into my lap and splutters and coughs right in my face.

Thank you very much, I was waiting for that. Well, not really. Aidan has apparently not yet learned to put his hand in front of his mouth when coughing. After clarifying the exact symptoms, I examine the young man. His temperature is normal at 37.4; the paracetamol he received at eight will have worn off by now. Aidan has a snotty nose, his throat appears normal as are his ears and the glands in Aidan's neck are only mildly swollen. A listen to the chest brings no further abnormalities to light.

Now I look at the offending eye, it is watery, not red and there is no pussy discharge. All symptoms point to a diagnosis of the common cold and I explain this to grandma. After advising her to return if his symptoms worsen or don't improve, Aidan waves and skips out of the door, waving his toy car through the air as though it's a plane.

* * *

It is one! This means that my on-call is officially over, even if I still have things left to take care of. At least no further ring-backs should arrive for me now. This current ring-back should, therefore, be the last one for today.

Seventy-eight-year-old Morris phoned to request dressings for his leg ulcer. Morris informed the receptionist that the district nurse asked him to do so. In general, it is the district nurse who will request these herself or even write the prescription herself, and I wonder why Morris is requesting the dressings himself. On the list are three dressings, all of which he has had prescribed in the last few weeks. I issue the prescription and send a task to inform the receptionists the prescription is ready.

Now I can get on with the remaining jobs on the list, knowing I won't get any further behind with my appointments.

* * *

This should be the last patient of today. Eighty-year-old Thomas attends with his wife, "Tom has had this rash for eight weeks. His cream is running out and we need another prescription. It works well for him."

So why did 111 consider it urgent for Thomas to visit the doctor today? This makes no sense to me.

"What cream does Tom use for his rash?"

Tom pulls out a small tube which is severely battered and bruised. The tube looks like the last little bit has been squeezed out of it. With difficulty, I can make out the writing on the label and I find this is hydrocortisone cream, a mild steroid cream, "How do you use this cream?"

Tom explains that only if his eczema is as bad as it now is, he will use the cream on the worst affected areas. At this time, he will use a tiny amount and use the cream sparingly for as short a period as possible to control his rash. Once the eczema is under control again, he only uses the moisturiser.

Brilliant! Thomas knows how to use the cream appropriately and thus reassured, I issue another prescription of the cream. Another happy customer.

* * *

When I close Thomas' notes and return to the appointment screen, I find another ring-back on the list. Strange. No more ring-backs should have been added after one, and I wonder if the receptionist has done so in error. Perhaps she did not realise I was only on call in the morning. She should know, though, I don't work on a Friday afternoon.

When I read the notes, it appears this has come in before one, the timestamp of the entry reads 12.59. This ring-back was for me after all.

A nursing home is requesting a prescription for dressings for one of their residents. Unfortunately, the dressings they ask for are difficult to find and it takes ten minutes before I find them all and can sign the prescription. A task to inform the receptionists follows.

* * *

The remaining ring-backs have 'urine sample' written next to them. Linda, our healthcare assistant, added them after she tested the urine samples.

The first result is from fifty-four-year-old Valerie who recently underwent bladder surgery and believes she has a urine infection. Other than a microscopic trace of blood, the urine sample is clear and I send a task to inform Valerie of this and advise her to repeat the sample again early next week. The blood in her

DIARY OF A FEMALE GP

urine is most likely because of the recent surgery, but we don't want to miss anything.

* * *

The next sample is from thirty-four-year-old Emily, the lady who phoned to ask for antibiotics for a urine infection. The details she has added when she handed in the sample include that Emily is pregnant. This will influence which antibiotics we can prescribe if she indeed has an infection.

The sample contains nitrites (a substance produced by bacteria and evidence of bacteria in the urine), leucocytes (white blood cells which fight infection) and a trace of protein. This suggests a urine infection and antibiotics are advised. After double-checking her notes and confirming she is not known with any allergies, I prescribe amoxicillin and send a task to the receptionists to inform Emily of this.

* * *

The next sample is from seventy-six-year-old Gerald, who has recently had prostate surgery. Gerald complains of pain on passing urine, not an unusual problem after this type of surgery and his surgery was only a week ago. Other than the presence of blood, his urine sample is normal. As the blood is not unexpected under the circumstances, I request Gerald to repeat the urine sample in a week.

* * *

The fourth urine sample, and after this one there is only one more left, is from five-year-old Aimee. Over the last week, Aimee has been bedwetting, and she was previously dry during the night. Mum wonders if she suffers from a urine infection and has brought in a sample to have this excluded.
Bedwetting is not considered abnormal unless it persists past the age of seven. As Aimee is only five, we can consider this to be within the normal limits. However, Aimee was dry during the night until last night and this might point towards an infection or an emotional upset. When I check the results, the urine is clear. Not an infection in that case. I send a task to inform mum of the results and to advise her to make an appointment with a doctor in routine if the problem persists. Could there be another reason behind Aimee's bedwetting?

* * *

The last urine sample waiting on my list is from

twenty-eight-year-old Simon. His symptoms are painful urination and a penile discharge. The urine sample he brought in appeared to be clear, though. As this is a rather sensitive problem and could point towards a sexually transmitted disease, I decide to phone the patient rather than send a task.

"Hi, is that Simon?" He confirms this. "Can you talk at the moment?"

"Hang on a moment doctor, I'll move to a quieter area." In the background I hear footsteps, a door opening and closing and then it is a little more quiet. "I'm in the photocopier room at the moment, we can talk."

When I explain about his clear urine sample and ask about the discharge, Simon admits he had unprotected sex two weeks ago.

"Okay, I think you should book an appointment at the GU clinic at the hospital. You can book this appointment yourself and don't need a referral from the doctor for this. These appointments are very private and they only send information to your GP if you request them to, otherwise not even we learn about your attendance." The GU clinic is short for genito-urinary clinic and they deal with sexually transmitted diseases mainly. Simon makes noises of agreement at the other end of the phone.

"From your symptoms and what you have told me, it is possible you have a sexually transmitted disease. In that case it is also important to perform contact tracing and the GU clinic is good at doing that. Are you okay with that?"

Simon agrees and we finish the call after he thanks me for the advice given.

CHAPTER 32

Friday, 1:25 pm

By now it is twenty-five past one and the pressure continues to build. I will need to leave the village by half-past two at the latest if I want to get any chance of getting to school on time. With a bursting bladder, I go upstairs to check the mailbox and any prescriptions still waiting for me in the office.

Libby calls me over, "Can you sign a few prescriptions while you are here?" and Patricia joins in, "There are a few forms I need you to sign too."

Not much chance of any extras right now, "Sorry girls, I need to rush, I still have lots of paperwork waiting for me downstairs, two visits to do and I need to get to school in time for Alex too."

Patricia pulls back the forms, "Don't worry about these, they can wait. I'll put them in your box instead."

After a quick bathroom break, I pass the practice manager's room, "Oh, Dr Ellen, can I have a word, please?"

What will it be this time? Not another complaint, I hope. I walk in, "What is the problem? I don't have a lot of time, there are still two visits to do before picking my son up and I need to finish more paperwork before I leave too."

Angela pulls out a letter, "This is important."

Not another complaint, please.

"This is the response from the defence organisation on your response to the complaint earlier this week. They approved your letter. Would you like me to send it for you?"

The sooner we finalise this problem, the better, "Yes, please."

After signing the final letter Angela has printed off, I wish her a good weekend and return to my room. At least there was not an extra worry piled on top of all the others.

* * *

A box with prescriptions is waiting for me when I enter my room. All prescriptions will need signing before I leave today; I won't be back until Tuesday and that would bring the processing time to over forty-eight hours. I take the prescriptions out of the box and place them in front of me on the desk. There is no time left to spend on unnecessary tasks or things I can also do at home; I will need to prioritise what is necessary and what can wait. At twenty-five to two, I only have ten minutes if I want to allow enough time for the visits.

One hundred and fifty-six electronic prescriptions are waiting. They can wait longer since I can also sign those at home.

One hundred and seven results are waiting. This will take too long and I can check them at home.

Any notification received can also wait until later to read and deal with.

There are one hundred and fifty-nine tasks in the task list at the moment, forty-five miscellaneous, which I can probably sort out at home. Forty-three repeat prescriptions for review and reauthorisation, they can wait until later too. Twenty-three labelled 'for information only'. There is definitely no rush with those. The forty-eight acute prescription requests cannot wait until I am home or until after the weekend. Hopefully, ten minutes will be long enough to work through those, however, we allow a week to process these and if the worst comes to the worst, I can always finish those later.

While I work my way through the list of prescription requests, I also sign the prescriptions in front of me. Every little moment in which the medical records take to load, I put to good use and sign a few prescriptions. When it is a quarter to two, I still have four prescription requests waiting and I decide to finish those before leaving for my visits.

* * *

As soon as the last prescription prints and the computer switches off, I grab my bags, sign the prescription and add it to the other signed prescriptions in the box in front of me and grab a box with medical notes to process this weekend. It is time to leave. On my way to the car, I drop off the prescriptions at reception, wish the girls a pleasant weekend and inform them I will be off to do my visits and home after that.

After I place the bags in the car boot, I make my way to the first visit. It will be a rush to make it in time for the school run.

* * *

The first visit is for ninety-six-year-old William, who lives in the nursing home. When I reach the home, I park, get my visit bag and ring the bell. It feels like hours before a nurse finally answers the door. In reality, it is probably only one or two minutes.

Although I realise they can't leave a resident to their own devices to answer the door, every brief delay seems to be too much today.

"Oh, doctor, who have you come to see?" the nurse asks in a cheery voice.

"Afternoon, I'm here to see William. I'm afraid I've not got a lot of time, there is another visit I need to do before picking my son up from school."

The nurse smiles at me, "No problem, we can be quick. William has picked up a little since we spoke to you. Although he still has a nasty cough, we are no longer as worried about him as we were before."

William had a stroke six months ago and ever since he has suffered from swallowing problems. This puts him at an increased risk of aspiration, inhaling his food or drink instead of swallowing it. And this puts him at an increased risk of chest infections.

After the nurse shows me his observations, his temperature mildly raised at 37.6 degrees, his pulse normal at eighty-five beats per minute and his oxygen levels at 96%, we enter William's room.

The nurse moves closer to the patient, "Afternoon William. This is Dr Ellen, is it okay if she has a listen to your chest?"

William cups his ear, "What?"

The nurse again repeats the question, this time a little

louder.

"You don't need to shout, you know, I can hear you perfectly well."

A smile tugs at my lips, and I try to suppress it. When I listen to William's chest, there is crackling on the right side as evidence of a chest infection. After explaining the findings to William and the nurse, I issue a prescription for antibiotics. Of course, after first making sure he has no allergies and can safely swallow the medication. Advice to seek medical attention if William's symptoms worsen or don't improve follows and I'm off to the next patient.

* * *

Now I drive over to Trevor's house. Trevor is only fifty-eight and terminally ill with bowel cancer. The district nurse believes he might not live beyond the weekend and requested a home visit for him today.

The foremost reason for this is to prevent unnecessary distress for the family. In the medical world, there is something we call the two-week-rule. If a patient dies, and if a doctor has not seen him within the last two weeks of life, the coroner needs to be consulted. This may mean that a post-mortem examination will take place, even if it concerns an expected death due to a pre-existing illness. If, however, a doctor has seen the patient within those two weeks, the doctor can issue a death certificate as long as the doctor is satisfied as to the cause of death and that no foul play is behind this death.

Trevor was last seen a little over two weeks ago by one of my colleagues. I have not seen him for quite some time and when I enter the living room, I'm shocked at what I find.

Trevor always was a rather plump person, not quite obese, but certainly overweight. Today he resembles a skeleton; you can count his ribs, and the jawbones are protruding. I can hardly recognise him.

Trevor meets my eyes with his sunken ones and smiles, "Nice to see you, doc, not seen you for a long time."

"Yes, you are right, it must have been a few years since I last met you. How are you holding up today?"

Trevor points to the syringe-driver, "Much better since you increased the pain relief, thank you. Managing okay now."

We chat a while longer and he tells me how it won't be long now, "I can feel it in my bones."

Trevor's wife, his two daughters and a son-in-law sit around his bed. Mary, his wife, wipes away the tears from her eyes and one of his daughters wraps an arm around her, "It will be okay mum," while handing her a hanky.

Even with the pressure of needing to leave soon, I make sure to give the impression I have all the time in the world for Trevor. This may very well be the last time I will see him alive. I agree with the district nurse, I don't expect him to last the weekend. At twenty-five past two, I get up and say goodbye to Trevor.

Mary and her daughters take me to the side when I leave, "How long do you think he has left? Should we ask Bill to come over from America?"

Bill is their son and if he wishes to be here before his father dies, he should be quick. How can I word this? "I can't really say how long it will be. Anything I say is only a guess, and Trevor may surprise us. My gut tells me this is a matter of days, but as I said, he may surprise us."

The eldest daughter meets my gaze, "Thank you, doctor for being frank, I will phone him as soon as you have left."

There are a few more practicalities to be discussed. One is the fact that I'm not here until Tuesday and if he were to pass away before then, this would be the earliest I could sign the death certificate. Sometimes, the out-of-hours service will advise the family to collect the certificate at ten the next morning. This only adds to the distress for the family and I would like to avoid that. I wish them luck and strength in the days and weeks to follow and offer them support if they need it.

Now it is time for me to leave and make my way to school to pick Alex up. I hope I will make it in time.

CHAPTER 33

Friday, 2:28 pm

As is to be expected, the journey home is riddled with delays. The motorway is rather slow today, and I wonder if there has been an accident. I hear nothing about an accident on the radio though and the signs along the motorway don't inform me of this either. Just the blinking fifty sign in the middle reservation. Not that anyone will drive any faster than that at the moment. A glance at my speedometer tells me I'm doing thirty at the most, but often less than that.

After fifteen minutes of this slow pace, the flow of traffic picks up a little. Although I'm only doing fifty-five at the moment, it is better than it was. What time is it now? The clock in the car tells me it is ten to three already and there is still at least a twenty-minute drive to get to school. Hopefully, there won't be any delays once I leave the motorway, but I have no guarantees and very little hope of that.

Once the traffic flows smoothly again, some idiots overtake at a speed far above the speed limit. Not the best of a plan when it is foggy like today and I hope they won't cause an accident and further delays. The urge to tap the steering wheel impatiently is strong and instead, I tap it to the beat of the music. Perhaps this will help me relax a little and calm down the palpitating heartbeat. Still, my throat tightens a little as I worry I might not get to school in time. Come on everyone, drive sensibly and safely and stop being an idiot risking the lives of others and your own. I need to safely get to school in time.

When I take the exit from the motorway, luck seems to be with me. Initially. Before long I reach the end of the queue which will lead all the way to the roundabout. There is no way to avoid this queue as the only alternative route ends up at the same roundabout and is as busy as this one. I can see the queue of that one in the distance on the hill already.

Patiently, or perhaps not so patiently, I edge my way forwards as the traffic allows. I keep glancing at the clock and the worry I might not make it on time increases.

Finally, I reach the roundabout and once I clear it, the rest of the journey is without delays. That is until I reach the parking lot. Not one space is left available, people have even double-parked. After I reverse out of the carpark, I try the one at the community centre instead. Even this carpark is full and when I check my clock again, it is already twenty-two past three. It is unlikely anyone will leave the carpark before school comes out.

Instead, I drive back the way I have come and to a street a little further away. There is a sports club here, which also has a parking lot. Fortunately, a few spaces are available here and I park the car. Now I have a run through the park to get to school, will I get there on time? Twenty-six past three already. There is no choice, I will need to run to get to school in time.

* * *

I reach school at twenty-nine past three and the first children are already waiting on the playground. Not Alex's class yet, but I recognise the teacher from the year above. Emily moves over, "Bad day?" I nod. "You look like you have been running."

Again, I nod, "Yes, the parking lot was full, so I had to drive back to the sports club and park there. I left work late and traffic was also against me. But at least it's the weekend." To make myself feel better, I add a smile. "So, how was your day?"

Emily tells me she had a nice quiet day at home, she does not work on a Friday, read a book and did housework.

Yes, those were the days. In the past, I had Fridays off too, but no longer.

"Any plans for the weekend?"

The plans for the weekend are not very exciting, "Nothing fun, I'm afraid. I need to work on an audit for work and get medical notes summarised, and, of course, I need to catch up on the housework."

Soon Alex runs up, "Mum, mum," he pulls on my sleeve and I pull my attention away from Emily, "can Christian come to play?" Christian is another friend of Alex's.

"Is that okay with Christian's mum?" Alex nods. "Then it's okay with me. We will need to talk to his mum first though."

Anna is okay with the plan the boys cooked up, "I'll pick him up at seven if that is okay." We say goodbye, Anna grabs Christian's school bag and Alex, Christian and I walk back to the car while Christian holds on to his football.

"Where are you going?" The direction I take confuses Alex, and he tries to pull me to the usual carpark.

"Sorry, we need to go this way today, there was nowhere to park today, so I had to use the parking lot at the sports club instead." The boys skip through the park and Christian kicks the football he brought with him. For a moment they play football on the grass together, then they run to catch up with me.

"What are we having for tea tonight?" Alex looks up at me, "Can we eat pizza tonight?"

Really? Again? We had pizza last night. "Shall we think of something different? You had pizza yesterday."

His face lights up, "Pancakes?" and his face falls again, "Oh we had that on Wednesday." A brief pause follows, "Can we have it again?"

Quickly I run it through in my head. Eggs? Yes, there are enough left. Flour? Yes, this is not a problem either. Milk? Yes, I got more when I went shopping last night. "Okay, we can make pancakes if you like. We'll make it full-sized ones today, okay?"

Alex's little face beams, "Oh, oh, can we have apple pancakes? And bacon ones? And ones with mushrooms?" His nose wrinkles, Alex does not like mushrooms, but Adam does.

After telling the boys they can have any pancake they like, we reach the car and soon we are on our way home again.

CHAPTER 34

Friday, 4:00 pm

When we arrive home, Alex dumps his bag at the front door and kicks off his shoes, Christian copies this and two pairs of shoes lie haphazardly in front of the front door. I pick them up and place them on the shoe rack; less risk of tripping over them. Alex and Christian run downstairs to the kitchen, and shortly after, I follow. They already have cups and pour squash in them. The boys can't reach the tap yet and I take over, "Here you go. Would you like a biscuit to go with that?" Of course, they don't decline the offer.

After they finish their drinks, they disappear upstairs to Alex's bedroom to play and I rush upstairs to change in jeans and a shirt, then return to the kitchen.

* * *

Now it is time for free time, or is it? No, not for me. It may be outside of office hours for me and time I don't get paid for, but more work is waiting for me. Once I have started the laptop and logged on to the clinical system, I first need to enter the details of the visits. It is always important to enter any details as soon as possible, but with Trevor's problem in mind, this is even more important today. Except for entering the details on the notes, I also do a letter for the Out-of-Hours service to make them aware of Trevor. This way they will be in a position to provide the best possible care to him if Trevor needs their help. A task follows to the receptionists to print this letter off and fax it to them. Good, this is completed and I can continue to the next job.

 The electronic prescriptions now take their turn, all one hundred and sixty-three. Wait, one hundred and six-three? I am certain there were less before. Someone must have added extra prescriptions to my list. The time stamp shows that Patricia added another seven prescriptions to my list at ten past two; after my day had officially ended. This could be an accident. They are prescriptions for a husband and wife, but still they are on my list.

 With the electronic prescriptions out of the way, I turn my attention to the tasks. One by one I tackle those; these also generate a few more prescriptions. The letters are next and I take care of the red-flagged first as usual, sending tasks to the receptionists as appropriate.

A message from Michelle pops up, "What do you think you are doing, creating more work for us? You shouldn't be working, you're supposed to be off. Shut down that laptop and relax."

As though that is at all possible, "Sorry, you know how it is, the work needs to be dealt with." Michelle knows; she has difficulty leaving a job unfinished herself but does not take work home with her. That is a drawback only the bosses or doctors have. Leaving a job undone can potentially harm a patient. However, we are only human and can only cope with a certain amount of work at a time.

Archie, Amy and Adam get home at five, as usual, they take their bags to their rooms and join me in the kitchen to grab a drink and a snack. Still the results to work through and I hope to get this done soon so I can start preparing tea.

Amy comes up to me, "What's for tea tonight?"

When I tell her they are having pancakes, she seems disappointed, "The big ones, what kind would you like today?"

Amy tells me she would like plain pancakes with syrup and Adam orders pancakes with apple, mushroom and bacon. Archie glances over when he hears that, "Oh, can I have those too?"

I continue work for a while longer, until the last result is filed away.

* * *

Half-past five already. With the work now out of the way, I put the laptop away and start tea. Soon the batter is ready, the mushrooms sliced and the apple cut in pieces. There were still unsmoked bacon lardons in the fridge too. The frying pans are on the stove, and I add a little oil. Just as I am ready to turn on the gas, I realise I have not asked Christian and Alex what pancakes they would like to eat. To find out, I move upstairs and ask them. Alex wants apple pancakes and Christian would like to try bacon. When I return downstairs, I prepare the requested pancakes, baking three at a time.

* * *

Soon the first pancakes are ready, and I call the kids to the table. Everyone enjoys their pancakes and Christian's second pancake is one with bacon and apple, "I've never had a pancake like this before, they are nice." While the kids eat their tea, I continue to make more pancakes, attempting to keep up with their demand. Their knives, forks and mouths work faster than I can prepare pancakes, but they will have to wait their turn.

I'm also watching the news and this is as depressing as always. When everyone only has room left for one more pancake, I offer to make this a dessert pancake, "How about making a pancake with a face? Eyes made of ice cream and chocolate drops, a nose made of a cherry and a mouth out of a piece of banana. We can use whipping cream for the hair and eyebrows. What do you think?"

Shouts sound all around me as the idea excites them. When the first ones are ready for Alex and Christian, Christian is quick to pick up his knife and fork again, but then drops them next to his plate again. Instead, he takes his mobile phone out of his pocket and snaps a picture, "I want to show this to my mum. Maybe she can make pancakes like this one day too."

Now all the batter is gone, and the kids finished their meal, the kids return to their bedrooms while I tidy everything away. I check the time and notice it is already a quarter past six, high time to make the preparations for our tea. Martin will probably be home around seven again. Today I have a treat for us, fresh mussels. Fries and peas will go well with that meal, but before I do anything, I will first need to clean and examine the mussels. All the mussels that won't close when tapped I put to the side, I remove all the surrounding debris, and place them in a mussels pan we bought in France on holiday last year. Chopped onion and oil are waiting on the bottom of the pan and once all the mussels are all in the pan, I add curry powder, parsley and chopped garlic. All set, they only need ten minutes and I'll wait until Martin is home before putting it on the stove.

At half-past six it is time to put the fries in the airfryer. They take about half an hour and that's when I expect Martin to be here. The peas can wait another ten minutes. And now the wait starts for Martin to come home and Anna to pick Christian up.

* * *

At ten to seven, I think it is safe to turn the peas on. It should not be much longer until Martin gets home. The fries only need a short while longer, but I will leave the mussels until he is here. When the bell rings at around seven, I turn down the flame under the peas and go upstairs to open the front door, "Hi, I'm here to pick up Christian as promised. Has he been good? Not caused you any problems?"

I assure her Christian has been an absolute angel, in fact, I have not seen or heard the boys other than at tea, "Let me get the boys for you."

When I reach Alex's room to inform the boys Anna is here, they are not pleased. "Ah, already? That's not fair. Can Christian stay for a sleep-over?"

"Not tonight, maybe another time. Christian's mum is here now and we don't want her to be here for nothing now, do we?"

Christian's eyes plead with me, "She won't mind, you can ask her."

"No, let's leave that for another time and we can plan ahead in that case and make sure you have all you need for the sleep-over with you."

Christian and Alex glance down, shuffling their feet, "Oh, okay then," and they shuffle down the stairs.

Anna notices the expression on the boy's faces, "Did you have a good time?" They nod and then Christian's face brightens, "We had pancakes tonight," he pulls out his phone and shows Anna the picture, "look, we got face pancakes for afters. Can you make those for us too, please?"

When I face Anna, I mouth, "Sorry" to her. I really dropped her in it in my attempt at treating the boys.

Once Anna and Christian leave, I return to the kitchen to keep an eye on the stove while waiting for Martin to return home.

* * *

A glance at the clock confirms it is after seven. Why is Martin not home yet? This is not like him. I turn off the gas; the peas are ready. The fries will be ready in two minutes. My mobile phone announces a text and I read it, "Sorry, on a visit. Taking longer than expected. Have phoned for an ambulance and now waiting for it to arrive. Been told this can take a while as a GP is with the patient."

I answer Martin's text and switch the oven on. The fries and peas can stay there to keep warm and I'm glad I did not put the mussels on yet. Hopefully, the rest of the food won't be ruined by the time Martin gets home.

While I wait I watch the television and read a medical journal. Martin has promised to text when he leaves and I'll wait for that before completing the food preparations further.

* * *

When I reach for a second medical journal to read, Martin texts again, "Coming home now." It's half-past seven and the journey home takes half an hour. While keeping an eye on the time, I continue reading for a few more minutes. At quarter to eight, I put the mussels on. Martin won't be long now.

CHAPTER 35

Friday, 8:03 pm

Shortly after eight, the front door opens and Martin returns home. This has been an extremely long day for him. Today he left at around half-past five and his day finishes at eight. Or, hopefully, it will. Footsteps make their way upstairs as Martin bolts for our bedroom to change. I put on the mussels and join Martin upstairs. After a hug to show my support, he finishes changing into something more comfortable.

"That was a long day, what happened?"

While we move downstairs to the kitchen, Martin's lunchbox in my hand, he tells me how he received a call for an urgent home visit at half-past five this evening, "This elderly man is known with COPD and his breathing was worse than normal. As his family suspected he might have a chest infection, they asked for a visit for their dad to be assessed and treated."

By now we reach the kitchen and I put the lunchbox in the dishwasher and turn my attention to the pan with mussels. After giving it a quick shake, I lift the lid to see how they are doing. Not all are open yet and I leave them for a while longer.

* * *

After another five minutes, the mussels are ready, and I put the food on the table.

Martin continues his story, "When I arrived, the patient appeared to have severe difficulties with his breathing and after assessing him it became clear, he should be in hospital and not at home. I then phoned for an emergency ambulance, gave them the details and informed them I felt he was unstable enough to require an emergency response. To my surprise, they informed me they did not class this as an emergency but merely urgent and as a doctor was present with the patient, it could take up to an hour before the ambulance would arrive. Absolutely ridiculous! They forced me to wait with the patient for over an hour as he was not stable enough to leave." Any other Friday, Martin would have left work at six after a long day, but not today. His colleague was on holiday, which meant he was on duty instead, "But, how was your day? Did you leave on time?" Martin faced me again, and I told him about my day at work while we enjoyed the mussels, peas and fries.

* * *

When we finish eating tea, we load the dishwasher and switch it on.

"I'm off upstairs to relax," Martin goes upstairs, while I load the washing machine with school uniforms and Martin's and my work clothes. With the housework out of the way, I join Martin in the living room.

Rather than relaxing as he mentioned, Martin has his work laptop in front of him and is entering the details of the visit in the patient's notes.

"I thought you said you were going to relax?"

"That was the plan, but I'll need to enter the details of the visit and I also have results and letters waiting for me." Next, he focuses his attention on said results and letters, while also watching the television. After another quarter of an hour, Martin closes his laptop and switches on the PlayStation, while I read my Kindle for a while. Now we finally have time to relax. The weekend has started.

* * *

Around half-past nine I get up and kiss Martin on the top of his head not to disturb him from the game, "I'm off upstairs, see you in a bit," and head for the bedroom. While Martin continues with the game, I get ready for bed and Martin follows half an hour later.

It has been a difficult and busy week with early starts, but this is not unlike many other weeks. Okay, with one colleague on holiday and one off for a morning because of illness, it has been more stressful than usual. Still, it could have been worse, and this week was not unusual.

Tomorrow will be Saturday and since we both don't work in the weekends, we should have a chance of a lie-in tomorrow. This promise lures me in until I realise the housework will still be there in the morning. And how could I forget? The audit and the summarising of records won't do the job for me on their own either. No, the envisioned lie-in will probably turn out to be a mirage. But for now, I can rest and sleep.

CHAPTER 36

Saturday, 6:55 am

Even without the alarm set, I still wake up before seven this Saturday morning. The habit of getting up early is by now so ingrained into the fibre of my being that even in the weekend I wake up early. Today is great. Sometimes I wake at five or six already. I turn over, but sleep does not return and at seven I get up and ready for the day ahead. There is plenty of work waiting, anyway.

* * *

Saturday is no different from any other day, I wash and dress and clean the bathrooms. The house still needs to be clean. Having three boys makes sure of that. When the bathrooms are clean, I trail to the kitchen to continue my tasks there. Indeed, no different to any other day of the week.

* * *

In the kitchen, I go through the usual daily tasks, measuring and mixing the dough. Today, I want to make baguettes and this means leaving the butter out of the recipe. I set the oven to 230 degrees rather than 220 and I add a tray in the bottom of the oven while it is heating. Sandwich baguettes are a special treat I make every so often.

The washing machine is unloaded, and I put the laundry in a basket which I take outside to hang on the washing line. The sun is out this morning, and there is a gentle breeze. Ideal for drying the laundry outside. Now the washing is drying, I clean the washing machine, the bin and the floor and return to the dough to knead it again.

The dishwasher is next, and I set the table for breakfast as I unpack it. I clean the worktops and the table, the stove and form the dough in baguettes which I leave to rest for another twenty minutes while getting yesterday's load of washing out of the dryer. While folding and ironing, I watch the breakfast news and run over everything that needs to doing today. The house is still quiet; the kids are still in their bedrooms and Martin enjoys a well-deserved lie-in. By the time it is half-past eight the ironing is finished, and the laundry is waiting in a basket to take upstairs and tidy away later. A glass of water in hand, I open the oven and pour the water in the tray at the bottom, then place the baguettes in the oven to bake for twenty minutes.

While I wait for the baguettes to get ready, I prepare the filling. First, I cut iceberg lettuce, then slice cheese and cut cucumber and tomato, while boiling some eggs. I place the cutting board with all on the table and also a peppermill. The mayonnaise can wait until the family comes downstairs.

* * *

Soon the baguettes are ready and I leave them to cool for a few minutes before placing them in a bowl on the table. Breakfast is ready and waiting for when the house and its residents wake up and I get myself another cup of tea while I wait.

I cherish this brief moment of calm and know it won't last long. Before long the rest of the family will wake up and interrupt my peace. While I listen to the birds whistling outside, I allow this to relax me before another busy day.

* * *

It is still quiet upstairs and I allow everyone to enjoy a lie-in this morning. Following my moment of recharging, I get out my laptop to check any new results, tasks or prescription requests that may have come in after I shut down the laptop yesterday. With those out of the way, I check the unassigned tasks. Reports from the Out-of-Hours Service arrive here too. Amongst these is a task from Out-of-Hours regarding two-year-old Jack, the boy I saw yesterday as an extra. His mum was concerned Jack had tonsillitis, but everything was fine when I examined him. I was not convinced mum believed me when I told her, and the contact with the Out-of-Hours service last night appears to confirm this.

As I read through their report, I notice how mum told them about Jack's severely sore throat, his massive tonsils and his sky-high temperature. All, of course, without the help of a thermometer. The Out-of-Hours service invited Jack and his mum for a reassessment and reached the same diagnosis I reached earlier in the day again. Since a few hours had passed since I saw him, Jack's condition could have changed, but it appears it was unchanged when he visited Out-of-Hours.

Okay, the basic work is out of the way. Not every weekend I will do this. After all, the weekend is time off and I am not expected to work or check results. Instead, the weekend should be time to spend with my family.

However, I also use the weekend to complete work I don't usually have time to do. An example of this work is to do audits to monitor and improve the quality of the care we provide to our patients. An audit is a short research we do on at least an annual basis. There can be more of those audits in one year. The audit I am working on at the moment relates to the care of the diabetics in the practice. The aim of the audit is to look into the diabetic control of diabetics diagnosed in a one-year period and whether any action was taken if the control was unsatisfactory.

To help me do this research, I run a search for type two diabetics diagnosed in the last year and then realise this will not give me the data to work with. After all, if we diagnosed someone with diabetes in the last month, this will not tell me if the results were acted on and changes in treatment took place and what the result of any changes was. So, instead I run a search for patients diagnosed in the period between two years ago and one year ago. I run the search, and it shows that eighty-four patients were diagnosed in this period.

Now the rest of the work starts. In the ideal world, 100% of the records for these patients should include the initial results and this is an appropriate standard to set. The next standard to decide on is which percentage would be appropriate for a re-test at three, six and twelve months following the diagnosis and I set 80% for this. In the ideal world this also would be 100%, but not all patients will follow the advice given.

From research, we know the first year following diagnosis is most important. Reaching a good control within this first year greatly reduces the risk of long-term complications of diabetes, and we obviously want the best possible for our patient group. A good diabetic control would be below 48 mmol/mol, and I set 50 as the cut-off where treatment should be intensified. Intensification should happen in at least 80% of the patients with a level above 50, I decide, and now I have set all the standards for the audit; I go through the notes of the eighty-four patients, one at a time, to search for the data required.

This is a long and boring job, but it needs to happen by hand. The clinical programme can do only the search for the new diabetics. When I find the required data, I enter them in a spreadsheet, NHS number in the first column to enable me to see which patient's notes I have processed already. In the eventual spreadsheet, I will remove this column to ensure patient confidentiality.

* * *

At half-past nine, I hear footsteps upstairs. By now, I have processed the notes of ten patients. I shut down the laptop and tidy it away, then lift the basket of laundry to take upstairs.

On the way back downstairs, I ask the kids and Martin to come downstairs for breakfast and they soon join me in the kitchen. Now, I place the mayonnaise on the table, make myself a cup of tea and Martin a coffee and wait for everyone to arrive.

* * *

Archie is the first to enter the kitchen, "We're having baguettes?" His eyes twinkle as the skin around them crinkles.

Next is Adam, "Oh, yummy, baguettes," and he grabs one from the bowl and cuts it open. Amy and Alex follow, and they join us at the table and quietly prepare their sandwiches. When Martin joins us, the kids are already digging into their sandwiches.

"I missed you when I woke up. Why did you get up so early?" Martin looks at me with puppy-dog eyes and I nearly feel guilty for having left the bed at seven.

"Sorry, I woke at half-past six and by seven I had really had enough. Lots of work to be done, and I got up instead to make a start on that. Did you sleep alright?"

Martin nods, "I prefer to wake up with you next to me, though."

Amy looks from Martin to me, "Oh, yuk, will you two cut it out already?"

After eating our baguettes, we tidy up, Martin returns upstairs to read medical journals or do an online course and I return to work again.

* * *

Now I grab the vacuum cleaner and take it around the house. Everyone is awake now, so I should not get too many complaints. Unfortunately, I will need to work around everyone, avoiding legs and feet and getting in all kinds of awkward positions to reach places without touching the kids and Martin. They are all busy completing their homework or playing on their computers.

* * *

When I return to the kitchen, I notice the sky looks rather grey as though it is threatening to rain. Perhaps I should check on the laundry to see if it is dry yet. It would be a pity if everything got dry again after having dried.

Except for a few underpants and a handkerchief, the

laundry is not quite dry yet and I need to keep a close eye on the weather to ensure the clothes don't get wetter than they are already.

* * *

After turning the laptop on again, I return to work on the audit. Again this is a slow process and when I finish with a set of notes, I look up and check the sky. Half an hour after I started, the sky appears to clear a little. A watery sun peeks through the clouds, and I continue the work.

Now I open the fifteenth set of notes. Date of diagnosis entered on the spreadsheet. HbA1c (the diabetic control figure) recorded at the time of diagnosis? Yes. I note down the result in the spreadsheet next. The result was 52 and I search through the notes to find out if any action was taken and what that action entailed. The action taken consisted of dietary advice and education and advice to repeat the HbA1c after three months.

Had the HbA1c been repeated three months after diagnosis? No, but a repeated value is present in the notes four months after diagnosis. This is acceptable and can be put down as a pass. The result at this time was 46, which is good. Was any action taken following this result? Again I search through the notes and find a request for a repeat test to take place after another three months. This result was again good at 45 and the HbA1c was repeated at one year after the diagnosis. At this time the diabetic control had worsened to 56, and the patient started on medication. I enter all the details on the spreadsheet and continue to the next patient's notes.

By the time I have had enough of this, the numbers are swimming before my eyes and I am at risk of making errors; it is half-past twelve, and I have processed another thirty medical notes. Not bad for a two-hour period.

* * *

Now I decide I have done enough work for today and I turn off the laptop. Saturday is one of my days off, after all. Strolling outside to check the laundry, I find the clothes are dry and take them down. After placing them in the utility room to fold and iron later, I set the dining table and ask Martin and the kids to join me to eat lunch.

CHAPTER 37

Saturday, 12:30 pm

While we eat lunch, we discuss what homework the kids will need to do this weekend. It is the usual thing every weekend.

Archie turns towards me, "I only need to do my maths homework and then I'll be ready."

Amy agrees, "Yes, I have done most of the homework during the week already." She is the studious one, the one who is always preparing flash-cards and doing the homework at the first opportunity. Well, most of the time.

Adam grumbles something only and I realise he won't tell anything more about it. Pushing him on the subject will only lead to more trouble and I leave it for now and will raise the subject at a different time when we are alone. That way dramas may be prevented. He hates being asked about what he needs to do and much prefers to play games. Hopefully, he will soon get his act together.

Alex has to do a little maths homework too, and it

appears the kids will enjoy plenty of free time this weekend. But isn't that how it should be? After a long week of work, we should be able to relax.

* * *

After lunch, I tidy up again while the kids go upstairs to do their remaining homework, read a book or play on the computer or PlayStation. Martin returns to his studies and for me, it is time to get the lawnmower and mow the lawn. We have a sizeable garden and as the job of mowing the lawn takes around two hours; I have to take advantage of the dry and sunny weather today.

Usually, I start in the front, and I do so today too. The garden is on a slope and this means it is also a physically challenging job. I take the stairs to the back garden when the front is finished and continue the work there. Many times I need to stop and empty the lawnmower into the composting bins at the back of the garden. But, before I can mow the lawn at the back, I first need to pick up any fallen apples and put those in the composting bins.

Phew, the job is done, I'm sweaty and my hands are green while leaves and grass stick in my hair. Still, my job is not done. The lawnmower needs to return to the garage, and the weeds need to be removed from the flowerbeds.

Two and a half hours after starting, the garden is finally looking like a garden instead of a jungle. Although I love gardening, there is simply not enough free time in my life to keep the garden under some semblance of control.

* * *

Now the job is finished, I make my way to the shower. I both need and deserve a shower after the hard work. Grass, leaves and little sticks fall from my hair and in the basin of the shower cubicle. The water cascades over my body as I allow it to soothe my now sore muscles. This week was my turn to do the lawn, next week it might be Martin's turn. Whoever has a chance to mow the lawn does.

After the shower, I change into clean clothes and return downstairs.

* * *

Back downstairs, I place the towels and my dirty clothes in the laundry basket and get my personal laptop out. Now it is time to relax. Relaxation for me consists of crafting, and making cards. As part of this hobby, I am also part of a design team for a crafting blog. Before I get my crafting supplies out, I read all my personal and crafting related e-mails, consult my spreadsheets and order any digital stamps from our sponsors for our team to use. Today I don't have a lot of time to work on this; it is nearly four already and with the planned meal; I realise I will need to start preparing it soon. Preparing Chinese takes a long time.

* * *

At half-past four, I shut down the computer and put it away. Today Chinese is on the menu and this means I need to make a lot of preparations. These preparations start with setting the table for our meal.

First, I break three eggs for an omelette, adding parsley and pepper. While that is frying, I cut an onion for the satay sauce I make.

The omelette is ready, and I put it to the side, taking out a pan and frying the onions until they are soft. Then I add a small jar of crunchy peanut butter and stir it until it is mixed. Now, I add ground ginger, coriander, garlic powder, cumin, curry and turmeric. I take a jar of sambal oelek from the fridge, this is a chilli pepper paste, and add two teaspoons to the mixture and now also add three teaspoons of soft brown sugar. The mixture needs stirring for a while longer before I add milk until a smooth paste emerges.

It won't be long before the satay sauce is ready and I add a little soy and leave it to heat a while longer before putting it to the side.

The next job is to put a large pan of water on the stove and bring it to the boil. Once it boils, I will add one nest of medium egg noodles per person to the water and allow it to soften and get ready. But in the meantime, I have a chance to cut the remaining ingredients for the bami goreng, which is like egg fried noodles.

Starting with spring onions, I cut those in thin slices, next I cut a carrot in small cubes. A small pack of cooked ham is cut in small squares too and the omelette is now cut in small strips. After placing the noodles to the side, I turn my attention to marinading the chicken for the satay. The marinade I use consists of soy sauce, cumin, coriander, garlic, turmeric, curry, ginger and sambal. I cut the chicken breasts into small cubes and stir these into the marinade to fully cover them and then leave the chicken for ten minutes.

Now, I get another three eggs and get them ready for a second omelette. This omelette will be egg foo yung. The version I make is called foo yung hai, which is the same in a tomato sauce. For the omelette, I also need a filling and I cut two more spring onions, a few button mushrooms and place them in a bowl. Cold water prawns will also be added when I prepare the omelette later on.

The tomato sauce is easy to make. I put one mug of bouillon in a pan and bring this to the boil, then add four tablespoons of tomato ketchup and next; I add ginger powder, cumin and a little garlic powder and a teaspoon of sambal. Again three teaspoons of soft brown sugar go into this too and this is mixed until a smooth sauce appears. However, it is still rather thin by now and to bind it, two teaspoons of cornflour are mixed with a little water and then poured and stirred into the sauce until it thickens. This I put to the side too.

The preparation stages of the food are now complete and I can start cooking the meal. I place the satay sauce and tomato sauce on two smaller burners and put them on a low heat, stirring occasionally. Two woks are added to the larger burners and with oil added, I fry the marinated chicken on a medium heat. To the other wok I add the cut spring onions, carrots, ham and omelette and also some petit pois. On top of this, I add cumin, coriander, garlic, turmeric, curry, ginger and sambal and I stir-fry this for a few minutes. After draining the noodles, I add these to the mixture and continue to stir-fry the mix. The satay is not forgotten about and I stir-fry this at the same time.

Once the bami goreng (egg fried noodles) are ready, I place the wok on the table ready for the family. It will remain hot for long enough to allow me to use the now vacant burner to prepare the foo yung hai. To do this, I first fry the spring onions, mushrooms and cold water prawns and add a little pepper and parsley. When they are ready, I place them to the side and prepare the omelette, adding the mixture to it while the egg is not yet set. Once this is ready, I fold over the omelette and place it in a serving bowl, then pour the tomato sauce over it. The satay sauce and the satay meat, I leave this in separate pieces these days rather than placing them on a skewer, also are added to the table, and it is time to call the family to the kitchen. My stomach is rumbling already.

CHAPTER 38

Saturday, 5:55 pm

Soon we are all at the table and enjoying the meal. Before long, Alex has his plate cleared and wants a second helping. He is mad about noodles and could eat Chinese every day if we let him.

Adam gets up and gets a glass of milk, "You've made it too spicy again." His eyes narrow and he stomps his feet as he strides towards the fridge. Everyone likes it spicy but Adam.

Martin and Archie go for second helpings too and I help myself to more too. Seeing how much the family enjoys the meal, makes it worth the effort of preparing it. Yes, we all love Chinese. Before long the food is finished, and we put everything in the dishwasher. Today no one has room left for dessert and they return upstairs while I continue to rinse the plates before stacking them in the dishwasher and turning it on.

* * *

With the dishwasher working on the dishes, I clean the table and worktop and wash a few dishes by hand. When I prepare Chinese, I use too many pans to fit them all in the dishwasher at once and only two choices remain. Either I wash them by hand, or I wait until the next day to put them in the dishwasher then. Tonight I might as well get rid of them and save myself time in the morning.

* * *

Now all the work in the kitchen is sorted, I walk upstairs and join the family in the living room for a quiet night together. Martin looks up, "I thought you would never get here. What took you so long?" and he points next to him on the couch indicating he wants me to sit there. As I sit down, he puts his arm around my shoulder and pulls me close, "That was a fabulous meal again, thank you," and places a kiss on my cheek. Together, we watch the news. All is set for a nice and relaxing evening. After a week of hard work, this is what we deserve and need.

* * *

After the youngest three have gone to bed, only Archie, Martin, and I are left in the living room and we decide to see a movie together.

"What would you like to watch?" Martin looks at me expectantly.

"How about one of the James Bond movies?" Archie and Martin agree, and we are soon enjoying the movie.

Midway through the movie, Martin turns towards me, "Can you get some crisps?" I nod and get up. Martin tilts his head to one side a little, "Maybe you can get me a drink when you are going downstairs anyway," and shows me his puppy-dog eyes.

A smile tugs at my lips and I promise to grab him a drink too, "What would you like?" then turn towards Archie, "Would you like a drink too?"

Soon I return with crisps and drinks for the three of us and we continue watching the movie.

* * *

When the movie finishes at just after nine, Archie leaves for his bedroom.

"How about a board game?" Martin turns towards me, "We could play Triominos or Monopoly or perhaps Scrabble." There is a question in his eyes.

Although it is a pleasant way to spend an evening together, the problem is he always wins. Well, maybe not always, but nearly always. And when strategy is involved in the game, I have no chance of winning at all. To lose one game is acceptable, losing more than one game and especially if it is three or four games in a row, gets very annoying.

Tonight is no different from usual. After Martin has won three games of Triominos in a row, we call it a night and go upstairs to bed.

* * *

As we go upstairs, my eyes start to close already. The week of work has worn me out and I am desperate to recharge. There is only one more day left of the weekend and not much chance to recharge. Weekends always seem too short.

Although I expect to fall asleep as soon as my head hits the pillow, the truth is different. My night is a disturbed one as thoughts of what needs doing the next day continuously enter my mind and keep me awake. Why doesn't work leave me alone at night?

CHAPTER 39

Sunday, 6:00 am

Six o'clock on Sunday morning. The warmth of my bed calls to me to stay in bed but my Fitbit buzzes me awake, and it is time to get up and complete more housework and also work on the audit again. After slipping out of bed and grabbing my bag, I slip to the bathroom to start another day. A yawn escapes and I would have much rather stayed in my warm bed and snuggled up to Martin.

* * *

The weekend is no reason to neglect the bathrooms and again I clean them. A daily chore which makes me realise I may not be too bad a housewife after all. The continuously putting myself down is a left-over from my youth. My dad was a person who did not believe in women developing a career, and many a time he would tell me I would never amount to anything, and I would never measure up. Becoming a GP against the odds has probably proven him wrong. Dad also believed a woman's first job was to do the housework, look after her husband and her family, and if you wished to have a career, do the housework too. The funny thing was, he never enforced that on my mum. Mum started a career when I was a teenager, and instead it was my job to do the housework according to dad as Mum was too busy.

This plays through my mind as I clean the bathrooms. I remember how Dad would come home around five or half-past five in the evening and sit and watch television. Every morning I would leave around half-past six after having done the housework and walking the dog, and I would return home around seven in the evening. After a long day at the university, the first thing Dad would say when I returned home was "Shouldn't you get started on preparing tea? Your mum will be home soon." No "Hello, how was your day?" No, my job was to get back to the housework as soon as I got home.

Although it is something I don't agree with in the slightest, it is something that has stayed with me my entire life and I still feel the urge and obligation to ensure I do the housework and everything related to my career as a GP too. One day I should consider myself to be 'good enough' but I'm not convinced that day will ever arrive. It's also one reason I can identify with people who are bullied in their career or at home so much.

* * *

The bathrooms are clean again, and I walk downstairs to prepare the bread. As I know I still need to do a lot of work on the audit and summarise several medical notes, I prepare bread rolls again today. Bread rolls are quick and easy to make and other than the kneading; they take little time. While the dough rests, I unpack the dishwasher, clean the kitchen, the bin and the washing machine and fold and iron the clothes. The entire job takes me around an hour and then it is time to place the bread rolls in the oven.

* * *

Now I get my laptop out again and check the results and the online prescription requests that have come in. Once I have dealt with these, I check the other tasks and notice a message from the district nurse. Trevor, the terminally ill patient I visited on Friday afternoon, has passed away. As I open his notes, I find out his son managed to come over from America just in time. A sigh of relief escapes. The opportunity to say goodbye can mean so much in the grieving process of a person. At the same time, my heart squeezes at the realisation Trevor is no longer with us, but at least he no longer suffers either. He was such a lovely man. The first thing I will need to do on Tuesday will be to sort out Trevor's death certificate. Hopefully, the Out-of-Hours service has not raised any unrealistic expectations. In the past, they sometimes informed relatives they could collect the death certificate at ten in the morning the next day. This is something which is not always possible. Still, they occasionally still tell relatives they can. At least I pre-warned the relatives on Friday and this may help them. Even though in these circumstances memories of what I told them may completely be forgotten.

I put my feelings over Trevor's passing to the side and get back to checking records for my audit. After processing ten more records, the oven beeps and I take the bread out of the oven. It is difficult to resist the smell of fresh bread and wait until everyone is awake before eating breakfast.

* * *

Putting the audit to the side for the moment, I move on to summarise several sets of notes. Every day new patients join the practice, and every day old patients leave. They move into the practice area, or they move away from it. To serve our patients best, we need to know all the important things about them. Any major illnesses they suffered with or they suffer from still. Any surgery the patient has had. If they have any allergies to medication or substances. Any medication they take or did not tolerate. When a lady had her last cervical smear and should be invited for the next one. Whether a child is up to date with all vaccinations.

To be able to do this, I need to read through the notes of the patients. Some notes are really thin and have hardly anything in them, while other notes consist of multiple folders and can take an hour at a time. The old notes are the worst, it can be extremely difficult to work out a doctor's handwriting. I spend an hour on this and summarise the notes of five patients. Not a bad achievement at all. All the details are added to the electronic notes and this should help us provide safe care.

* * *

I stop summarising when noises reach me from upstairs around nine. From the creaking floorboards and squeaky doors I realise Martin, Adam and Alex are getting up. Archie's door also opens, and he runs upstairs. After tidying away the laptop and the medical records, I set the table ready for breakfast.

Our bedroom door opens and closes. Martin makes his way down the stairs. The doors all have their special squeak enabling me to tell them apart. Now I know Martin is coming downstairs, I turn the kettle on and put some coffee in his mug. Not long after, he saunters in, "You were gone again this morning," and he pulls a sad face.

After hugging him, I kiss him good morning, "Sorry, but at least the bread is ready, and I got more work done."

Martin's face clouds over, "It's not right you should have to work in the weekend. Others in the practice should summarise too. Why don't you get some summarisers to do the work for you?"

There is a very simple reason for that. Hiring more staff is expensive and something we can't afford. The other doctors would never approve of the expenses involved. And I agree with them. At the moment this is not something we can afford as a practice. Martin does not agree with that but it can't be changed and someone needs to do the work.

The boys come in and sit down at the table for breakfast. Only Amy is still upstairs, and I go up to call her down for breakfast too. Not long after, we eat our breakfast.

"So what are you all planning for today?" I glance around the table. Four blank stares meet my eyes.

Archie mumbles something while eating his bread roll. Something that probably meant he will play on his computer today. Martin wants to study this morning and relax afterwards and I realise I still have work waiting for me too.

Breakfast finishes, and everyone puts their plate in the dishwasher and moves upstairs or to their rooms.

* * *

After cleaning the table following breakfast, I grab the laundry basket, head for upstairs, and put everything in the wardrobes they belong in. A quick bathroom break and I make my way downstairs again and take the laundry basket to the utility room before getting my laptop out again. Time for the next round of work today.

* * *

Now it is time to summarise a few more notes. By now it is already half-past nine and I resolve to summarise notes until twelve. In this time I only process another ten sets of notes, one set alone taking me nearly an hour. The notes reveal this patient is a diabetic. Details of her last annual review needs adding to the electronic records and a new recall date needs to be set for the next annual review. She also suffers with asthma, the last asthma review took place over two years ago and the patient uses inhalers. This means she should be seen annually, she must have slipped the net or not attended for her review when requested. On the patient's notes, I set next month's date for the review and I send a task to the receptionist who sends out the letters for recalls to make her aware she will need to send the patient an invitation. The patient's last cervical smear was last year, and it was normal, she needs another smear in two years as she is under fifty years old. All these details I add to the electronic notes too. A history of hypertension, high blood pressure, is also recorded in the notes, an annual review for this is not obvious in the notes. Perhaps as this can be done at the same time as the diabetic check, anyway. The date I put for recall for the hypertension review is the same date as for the diabetic review. The same goes for the date for the patient's annual CHD (chronic heart disease) review; she suffered a heart attack two years ago.

When I finally put away the last set of notes for today, it is twelve. I'm pleased with myself for having managed fifteen sets of notes this weekend. Still, it is only a start. We have a bit of a backlog at the moment after a recent influx of new patients. Martin is correct in saying we need to get more people involved with the summarising. Perhaps we can train our staff up to do this for us and I mull this over for a while.

DIARY OF A FEMALE GP

CHAPTER 40

Sunday, 12:05 pm

Although I have now put away the work for today, I feel guilty for doing so. Perhaps I should complete more work this weekend. Should I go back to work after lunch after all?

No, it has been enough for this weekend and I would like to spend some time for me too. Still, sometimes I wonder if I even own the right to spend time on hobbies. And when I spend this time on them, it sometimes makes it seem I'm neglecting more important tasks. Neglecting the duties I have as a doctor, a wife, a mother, a housewife. On a Sunday afternoon, I rebel against these feelings and I craft and enjoying myself. Often I will also spend time on studying and reading medical journals. I need to stay up to date.

At twelve set the table. It is time for lunch. After calling everyone to the kitchen for lunch, we spend this time together. The kids still plan to do their own things and, although Amy sometimes joins me for crafting, she does not want to join me today.

* * *

With lunch behind us, I clear the table and get my personal laptop out. But before I do anything else, I should study a little. In our job it is important to keep up-to-date on new developments and keep knowledge fresh. As part of our yearly appraisal to ensure quality, we need to put in a minimum of fifty hours of study a year. Although fifty hours does not appear to be a lot from a distance, it can be very difficult to make it fit in our already busy schedules. Time is limited during the weekdays and even in the weekend it's difficult to find time in between the housework and the work I still do for the job at home.

This year I agreed to update my knowledge of COPD as part of the continuous personal professional development. First, I work through one course, which takes an hour and I work through another online course too, another hour of work.

Martin comes to the kitchen to grab himself a coffee, "You're not still working, are you?" he raises his eyebrows and faces me. "There should be no need to work all weekend and all week long. Don't let anyone take advantage of you like that." With a coffee in his hands, Martin returns upstairs again.

Next, I read two articles from online medical news and update my learning record for my annual appraisal. In this we need to write when we did what and summarise the course or article briefly. Next it is important to write what the impact of the course or article is on your current medical practice if any and why and attach any certificates a course may have earned you. It can be quite a struggle to keep on top of all of this with all the other duties I need to fulfil in my life. Even fitting in time to study can cause stress as I need to use every little bit of time I have available.

Relaxation is an afterthought. Perhaps we are simply not allowed to relax. But, without relaxation, we would burn out and become worse doctors. The only way to make everything fit in might be to get up earlier than I do already. This is not likely to work. If I get up earlier, I need to go to bed earlier. Or I would not catch enough sleep. And without sufficient sleep, I would be too tired and be at risk of making mistakes. Making mistakes in a GP's life means risking lives. And that's not a good thing. Not a good thing at all.

* * *

By now it is already three in the afternoon and I complete the work and study related tasks I had set myself for today. It is time to relax with some crafting and I realise I will have limited time to create anything. Before I start, I first check all private e-mails and the ones related to the crafting challenge I am part of. A few images have arrived for the design team and I email them to the team members who requested them.

With those out of the way, I check on our brief for the upcoming challenge. Our theme is Christmas and I get out my supplies and create a Christmas card. Using papers I designed myself, and an image from our sponsor which I colour in, I create a design for the Christmas challenge. I add a ribbon and brads, a sentiment I created and after sticking everything together the card is ready. Daylight is still here and I snap a picture for the challenge and upload it to the design team blog.

Now the project for the coming week is out of the way, I create a few Sympathy cards. When one of our patients passes away, we send the relatives a sympathy card to offer our support during their bereavement. Usually these cards are the ones I make by hand and add my own sympathy poem to. Although crafting is a hobby, it also keeps our stock of sympathy cards up. And we will need another one this week following Trevor's death.

After an hour of focused attention to card-making, I

feel more relaxed and put my supplies and laptop away. A minimum of one hour spent on crafting is what I set for myself. Although I sometimes question myself on my right to relax, I know I need to safeguard this time to ensure I continue to function to the best of my abilities.

* * *

When I look at the clock, I notice my hobby has taken up more time than I had expected. It is half-past four already. Time to make tea. Today I will prepare roast beef with potatoes, broccoli, peas and carrots. As it is the weekend, I have more time to spend on cooking and I don't mind putting in more of an effort.

After seasoning the meat, turn on the oven to 190 degrees. Then I fry the meat until it is brown on all sides. Next I place it into the oven and it is time to get the rest of the meal taken care of.

The potatoes are in the cupboard under the stairs and I get them and peel them. Next the broccoli and carrots are prepared and I add peas to the top layer of the steaming pan. The meat still has another half an hour to roast, and now I put the potatoes and vegetables on the stove. All I can do now is wait for the meal to cook.

To pass the time, I grab my Kindle and read while still monitoring the food.

* * *

At half-past five, tea is ready and I call the family to the table. Alex is excited, "Roast beef, yummy." His eyes sparkle.

Amy is not a fan, but the other boys love the meal. Martin is not overly excited by the idea of beef either. As we all eat the meal, I enquire if anyone has any requests for tea during the week.

Amy looks up, "Can we have lasagne?"

Although lasagne is a great idea, this is not a meal to cook on a workday. Lasagne is far too time consuming to prepare. "Sorry, I won't have enough time to cook it during the week. Perhaps we can do that next weekend?"

She nods, "Okay."

When I ask if anyone has any other ideas, no proper suggestions come up. Not an unusual occurrence.

Martin turns to me, "I'll leave it to you to decide sweetheart."

But that is not why I asked. Help from the family in coming up with a meal plan for the week ahead would be welcome. I like to maintain a variation in our diet, but I can only come up with so much in the way of ideas myself. The input from the family might bring other and perhaps even nicer ideas. Instead, it appears it will be another week of fish on Monday, pasta on

Tuesday, burgers or beef on Wednesday and pizza on Thursday. More variation would be nice.

* * *

After we finish the meal, I clean the table and turn the dishwasher on. Now I can also go upstairs to join the family in the living room. It is already six and I won't have a lot of time before I need to go to bed. A look at the clock tells me it is already a quarter past six and before long bedtime will come along again. For now, I grab my bag and a drink I join the family upstairs. Spending time with my family is valuable as I spend far too much time working.

* * *

When I join Martin and the kids in the living room, I reflect on the amount of time I spent with them this weekend. This was an extremely limited amount of time and it makes me feel guilty. These days I only meet them at breakfast and teatime. And only if I get home before they go to bed, I will see them at teatime.
Again the sensation that I am a neglectful mother and that I am doing them a disservice surfaces. Should I not put their needs first? But then, shouldn't I put my patient's needs first too? When I think about it, I

realise my kids, husband and patients always come first. The only person who is an afterthought is me. Not for my kids and husband, but for me. As long as they are all getting the attention they need, everything is as it should be. Or is it? Should I look after myself better, perhaps?

Fortunately, the kids seem happy and content. Sometimes they complain when I can't be there to do things, but generally the kids appear to be content with how everything is. All four of the children do well in school, make friends well and we are extremely lucky, the kids behave well too.

At the moment they are all absorbed in playing computer games. Martin is playing on the PlayStation and none of them appear to have noticed my entrance into the living room much. After taking a seat on the couch, I pick up the Kindle and read further in the book I was reading.

* * *

Soon it is half-past seven. Time to go upstairs and get ready for bed. Tomorrow will be another early day; I set my alarm for a quarter to four again, as always on a workday. At least I only need to work two hours tomorrow. I will fill the rest of the day with household chores, shopping and the school run. It will be the start of another week. The same old, same old. New patients, fresh problems, but more of the same, anyway. There will be more colds and sniffles, earaches, tummy aches, joint and skin problems.

Still, there is a variation in the problems which walk through our doors. This is the benefit of General Practice, to encounter a variety of problems and a variety of patients. You also care for entire families and watch them grow up and grow older. Which also means you see the same patients time and time again and they become your friends in a way. And when they get older, the inevitable will happen. Eventually the people you have cared for over the years will die and you lose a friend. Although we learn to not get too attached through time, this will bring the occasional tear to our eyes too and a squeezing of our hearts. We are not machines after all.

But now it is time to get upstairs, get changed and go to bed. I need to get enough sleep to be able to cope with the coming week.

EPILOGUE

Thoughts from the author

Surely the life of a GP must have gotten easier by now? If that is the thought crossing your mind, I'm afraid you're mistaken.

"But how about the promises the government made in recent years? 5000 extra GPs. That must have helped."

Again, you're mistaken. The government made this promise, one that should take place over several years. To be honest, I'm unsure where they will get the GPs from. So far, more and more GPs retire. Some retire early, like Dr Ellen did, some retire when they really can't go on any longer. Dr Ellen knows one GP still going strong who is well into his nineties. We expect many more GPs to retire over the coming years and the 5000 promised GPs may not be enough to cover those who are leaving. But where will those new GPs come from? It is difficult to see where they will find these GPs. Abroad? But wasn't that what Brexit was about? No longer recruiting from and allowing people to settle in the UK from abroad? Or is there some hidden lab where they are creating test tube GPs?

There have been voices raised about accelerated training. But how good would that training be? Would that still guarantee excellent care?

The honest answer is that I don't know what will happen or whether the government will deliver on their promises or whether the work pressures will continue to increase as they are now.

What I do know is that Martin, Dr Ellen's husband, is still working. His partner retired, leaving him the only partner in the practice and left to care for over six thousand patients. Martin has regular locums and a salaried doctor working for him. However, if one of the other doctors is ill, he will need to work harder to pick up the slack or even come in during his holiday. Only a few weeks ago, he needed to come into work every single day of his week holiday. This can't go on. Everyone needs some down-time to function properly. So far, he is doing well and coping admirably. But how long can this continue? How long will it remain safe to practise under this continuous pressure?

No one knows. I only recognise things need to improve if they expect primary care to continue to provide the best care to their patients. That is the thing which is most important to those working in primary care. Often they will neglect themselves to give their patients their all. We can only hope that more doctors become GPs and the government puts more help in place. Simply piling on more responsibilities and requirements onto GPs and not providing the resources needed to deal with these is not something which will work. At least, not in the long run.

I hope you have enjoyed this little peek behind the scenes into the life of one GP and please bear this in mind if you go to see your doctor and he or she runs a little behind schedule. Possibly your doctor has been dealing with a complex problem and it might be you who needs a little more time the next time you visit the GP.

* * *

I wrote the epilogue before COVID-19. The event of COVID-19 has changed life beyond anything we ever expected. And with it, life in General Practice has changed.

No longer can you ring the doctor for a face-to-face appointment. Instead, appointments take place over the phone or by video link. Only when a GP feels a clinical need for a face-to-face appointment exists, will they see the patient. And only then if the patient shows no symptoms of COVID.

Online triage systems are in place to help to reduce

the workload of the receptionists and all staff in the practice. Prescription requests need to be requested online if at all possible. The doctor electronically signs the prescriptions and sends them to a nominated pharmacy. We keep direct contact with patients to a minimum.

Over the next months, life will return to normal. But will it ever go back to how it was? I expect that is unlikely. Online triage, telephone and video consultations are here to stay. Face-to-face appointments will only take place if clinically indicated. All these changes should reduce wastage of time for patients and the GPs.

Just think about it. Is it really necessary to discuss all results face-to-face? Probably not. It doesn't need a 10-minute appointment to tell a patient all their blood results are normal. That could be a 2-minute phone call instead.

We don't know what life in General Practice will be like after COVID. But we know it will be changed. Life in general will be different from before. Maybe a better work-life balance and less pollution will result. Time will tell.

Joni Martins

ABOUT THE AUTHOR

Joni Martins was born in the Netherlands and now lives in the United Kingdom with her family. She is in her fifties and she has so far written and published five books in her 'Friends, family and love' series. Four are available in both English and Dutch, the last one only in English. The first book, Captive Love, was published in December 2017.

Joni has always loved writing, but only seriously took up this hobby during her year of retirement. She is now working again and her writing has subsequently taken a bit of a backseat.

Joni is working on the sixth book in the series, and also is editing a supernatural romantic murder mystery.

Diary of a Female GP is a non-fiction book based on real-life General Practice in the UK and started as a NaNoWriMo project in November 2018. It will be published in 2020.

Meet up with Joni on her blog (https://jonimartinsauthor.blogspot.co.uk/) and website (https://sites.google.com/view/jonimartins), on Twitter (@JoniMartins3), Facebook, Instagram and Pinterest. She would be happy to meet you there. The latest developments regarding her work can also be found there.

OTHER BOOKS BY THIS AUTHOR

<u>CAPTIVE LOVE</u>

First in the 'Family, friends and love' series.

Lydia wakes up in a dark and damp cellar. Where is she? How did she end up here? And why?

Sam has admired Lydia from afar his entire life but she never noticed him. Now she is in his home.

Will Lydia learn to love Sam? Or will she escape?

And what will her friends and family do when they find out she is missing?

<u>FREED LOVE (18+)</u>

Second book in the 'Friends, family and love' series.

Lydia is back at the cottage she shares with Rob, her best friend's big brother. However, everything feels awkward.

Rob has difficulty coping with his feelings for Lydia now they have changed. Can things go back to how they used to be?

And what will happen when Sam returns on the scene?

FREED LOVE (CENSORED)

Second book in the 'Friends, family and love' series.

Lydia is back at the cottage she shares with Rob, her best friend's big brother. However, everything feels awkward.

Rob has difficulty coping with his feelings for Lydia now they have changed. Can things go back to how they used to be?

And what will happen when Sam returns on the scene?

HIDDEN LOVE

Krista and Theo want to open their best friends' eyes to their mutual love. Why can't Lydia and Rob not see what is going on?

However, they also discover a love of their own. Wanting to make sure what they have is real, they keep their love hidden.

A moment of inattention leads to the discovery of their love. Can it survive when Theo's mother and sister oppose it so much?

LOST LOVE
Fourth book in the 'Friends, family and love' series.

Josie regrets her harsh words when Theo breaks up with Krista and spirals into depression and suicidal thoughts. How could she have done this to her brother?

Will Josie and Ronald be able to repair the damage done? Can they save Theo? Can Josie save her friendship with Krista?

HOLIDAY LOVE
Fifth book in the 'Friends, family and love' series.

Ronald can't accompany Freya on her camping holiday this year as Theo is off work due to depression and Joshua is already on holiday at the same time.

When Joshua arrives at the campsite in Brittany, he can't believe his eyes when he sees a familiar car parked in front of a tent.

Follow Freya and Joshua as they explore beautiful sites, picturesque villages and castles in Brittany.

GROWING LOVE

Sixth book in the 'Friends, family and love' series. (still in progress)

Even little surprises can make a large impact.

Follow Freya and Joshua as they encounter surprises on their way. How will they cope with their parents' objections?

This book is still in progress.

WAKE-UP CALL

A paranormal, romantic murder mystery. (still in progress)

Daryll wakes up and gets ready for work as usual.

Still, something feels different. Why is his secretary ignoring him? Certainly, he can't have upset her this much?

And then …. The scream!

Why is Alicia screaming? And why is she shaking … him?

DIARY OF A FEMALE GP

Take a look behind the scenes of UK General Practice before COVID-19.

Based on real-life, this book follows a week in the life of a female GP.

All cases discussed could have happened and are based on similar occurrences the author's friend encountered.